YOUR
Inner Physician
AND YOU

YOUR
Inner Physician
AND YOU

CranioSacral Therapy
AND
SomatoEmotional Release®

JOHN E. UPLEDGER, D.O., O.M.M.

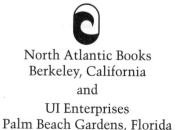

North Atlantic Books
Berkeley, California
and
UI Enterprises
Palm Beach Gardens, Florida

Your Inner Physician and You

Published by
North Atlantic Books
P.O. Box 12327
Berkeley, California 94712

and

UI Enterprises
11211 Prosperity Farms Road
Palm Beach Gardens, FL 33410

Cover and book design by Andrea DuFlon

Printed in the United States of America

Distributed to the book trade by Publishers Group West

Your Inner Physician and You is sponsored by the Society for the Study of Native Arts and Sciences, a nonprofit educational corporation whose goals are to develop an educational and crosscultural perspective linking various scientific, social, and artistic fields; to nurture a holistic view of arts, sciences, humanities, and healing; and to publish and distribute literature on the relationship of mind, body, and nature.

Library of Congress Cataloging-in-Publication Data

Upledger, John E., 1932–
    Your inner physician and you : CranioSacral therapy and somatoemotional release / John Upledger. — 2nd ed.
        p.   cm.
    ISBN 1-55643-246-1 (pbk.)
    1. Craniosacral therapy.   I. Title.
RZ399.C73U69   1997   96-37576
615.8'2--dc21   CIP

3   4   5   6   7   8   9 / 00   99

*This book is affectionately dedicated
to all those patients who have
kindly acted as guides and signposts
as I travel my path to today.*

*And to my big sister, Phyllis
who always helped me
through the rough spots.*

Dr. John

Contents

Introduction   xi

Preface   xiii

1   The Hook is Baited   1

2   I'm Hooked and Don't Know It   5

3   A Glimpse of the Core   9

4   I'm Hooked and I Know It   15

5   The Craniosacral System   17

6   Early Experiences with CranioSacral Therapy   20

7   The Horizons Broaden   29

8   Other Uses for CranioSacral Therapy   33

9   A Treatment for Depression   40

10   The Famous TMJ Syndrome   43

11   Chronic Pain and Disability   50

      Post-Herpetic Neuritis   51

      Crushed Pelvis with Severe Craniosacral
System Dysfunction   53

      Restoration of Brain Function After Coma   54

      Spinal Cord Injury   56

      Disability Prevention   58

12   Insights   62

13   Tissue Memory! What Next?   63

14   The Energy Cyst: A Model   71

15	Back to Tissue Memory and More	74
16	SomatoEmotional Release®	77
17	The Use of Healing Energy	93
18	Intention and Touch	101
	Sister Anne Brooks	102
	Coma Case History	106
19	Therapeutic Imagery and Dialoguesm	109
20	The Bottom Line	123
21	Who Can Do This Work?	125
22	The Anatomy of the Craniosacral System	130
23	How the Craniosacral System Evaluation and Treatment Are Carried Out	142
24	Other Areas of Application for CranioSacral Therapy	151
	Acute Systemic Infectious Conditions	151
	Localized Infections, Sprains, Strains, Bumps and Bruises	152
	Chronic Pain Syndrome	153
	Arthritis	153
	Emotional Disorders	153
	Scoliosis	154
	Ear Problems	154
	Cerebral Ischemic Episodes (small strokes)	154
	Visual Disturbances	155
25	Thank You CST-SER	156
	Multiple-Hands/Multiple-Therapists Treatment	157
	CST-SER and PTSD	160
	The Float Tank	164
	Getting Grounded	168
	When Divers Get Dizzy	172
	It's Music to His Back	175
	Working With Dolphins	177
	CranioSacral Therapy, Obstetrics and Pediatrics	184

The Brain Speaks   193
SomatoEmotional Release and the Psyche   197
Psychology and SomatoEmotional Release
by Russell A. Bourne, Jr., Ph.D.   197
How is SER Not Psychotherapy?
by John Page, D.O.   205
26 Questions & Answers   207
Closing   221

Illustrations

Illustration 1: Side view of spinal column showing
vertebra and discs 13

Illustration 2: Jamming of occiput (skull) into upper neck
(cervical) vertebra and how it can happen 22

Illustration 3: Temporal bone location in skull 26

Illustration 4: Top view of skull showing sutures and
location of Olivier's overlap between
frontal and left parietal bones 31

Illustration 5: The thoracic inlet release technique 61

Illustration 6: Direction and penetration of force as it
enters the body during a traumatic
experience 69

Illustration 7: V-spreading the eye .96

Illustration 8: Semi-closed hydraulic system of the cerebrospinal fluid and dural membrane 131

Illustration 9: Points of attachment of dura (detail) 133

Illustration 10: Back (posterior) view of sacrum and lower
spinal vertebra showing exit of spinal
nerve roots from within spinal canal 135

Illustration 11: Mechanics of dural sleeves, which allow
up-and-down movement of dural tube
within the spinal canal 137

Illustration 12: Experimental setup that demonstrates
movement of monkey skull bones 140

Illustration 13: Back (posterior) view of sacrum between
the ilia 145

Introduction

This book is about the discovery of a whole new body system—how it was found, where it has led and what it means to you. This newly discovered system has been named the craniosacral system.

This discovery offers you a chance at an improved quality of life no matter at what level you presently function. The use of CranioSacral Therapy and the more advanced techniques of SomatoEmotional Release® and Therapeutic Imagery and Dialogueˢᵐ to which it has led offers you, and everyone you know, the chance to realize new potential for healing and health enhancement on all levels.

This book provides for you a play-by-play, firsthand account of the development of this body of knowledge and the doors that it has opened in the use of body energies and self-healing.

In this new edition of *Your Inner Physician and You*, I have not tampered with the original text. This original text records the history of my own journey in the development of the concepts that relate to the craniosacral system and its uses as a modality of evaluation and treatment for patients and clients. This history has not changed and, as I reread this original text, I am satisfied that I have been faithful to the truth. Therefore, this original manuscript has not been changed.

Since that first writing, several things have happened which have caused us to implement a "certification" process for practitioners of CranioSacral Therapy. The stimuli that moved us to develop this certification process were several moves by healthcare professionals in several states to claim CranioSacral Therapy as a specialty within their own profession, and thus prevent other healthcare professionals from practicing it. In one sense, this was a compliment to Cranio-Sacral Therapy, because these people would only want control of something that held promise for them. On the other hand, if they did gain control of CranioSacral Therapy and who can practice it, many healthcare professionals from other professions would be excluded from the practice.

Originally, I put CranioSacral Therapy out there as an adjunctive modality that could be usefully and effectively incorporated in many kinds of healthcare practices, from massage to dentistry, and from physical medicine to body-mind integration. I still believe that this is its best use. However, the power moves and greed manifestations that have surfaced in several areas have made it clear that certification of Cranio-Sacral Therapy as an independent healthcare modality is essential in order to protect the rights of a wide scope of licensed healthcare professionals as they practice CranioSacral Therapy. This is simply a fact of life. And so we are certifying CranioSacral Therapists as such.

I have added a last chapter onto the text which presents and discusses several of the new and exciting things that have happened in the world of discovery. In these areas Cranio-Sacral Therapy deserves many accolades as it continues to open doors and offer introductions to new and innovative approaches to helping people heal.

Preface

Since the first writing of this book, a most exciting new chapter has begun to unfold. This unfolding has to do with the intensive and integrated uses of CranioSacral Therapy, Energy Cyst Release, SomatoEmotional Release®, and Therapeutic Imagery and Dialogue℠. The target problem which has presented itself is post-traumatic stress disorder.

The use of this integrated approach began to unfold in a variety of cases, such as the post-traumatic residual effects of attempted murders, rapes, satanic cult abuses, physical beatings, and the like. My own experiences, along with the reported experiences of others doing CranioSacral Therapy, began to stockpile. An inescapable question arose. Was CranioSacral Therapy, with all of its aforementioned offshoots, efficacious for what we call post-traumatic stress disorder? I decided to put it to the test.

We invited six Vietnam veterans to participate in a two-week intensive treatment program aimed at alleviating their post-traumatic stress disorder problems. Five of the veterans were men and had been in treatment for the sequelae of their problems for at least 10 years each. They all suffered from panic attacks, uncontrollable violent, explosive episodes, inability to concentrate, recurrent nightmares, uncontrolled sweats, and the like. In short, they were not able to pursue gainful employment or the development of meaningful careers, nor were they successful in establishing meaningful family relationships.

The sixth veteran was a woman who had spent two years as a front-line surgical hospital nurse. What she described was similar to the televised episodes of M*A*S*H. She suffered from nightmares, acute panic attacks, etc., but she managed to keep her problems secret and maintain a nursing position in a hospital.

I felt that if these veterans could experience significant improvement from a two-week intensive treatment program with us, this would be the acid test. As it turned out, the treatment program was more successful than we could have imagined. All six of the veterans demonstrated significant and ongoing improvement. The release of retained traumatic energy seemed to be the key factor.

We look forward to the continued refinement and development of this approach to alleviating the residual effects of severely traumatic life experiences.

1

The Hook is Baited

It was about 8:00 a.m. when Judy called me at home. She sounded really upset, trying hard to be calm, but her near panic was coming right through the telephone at me. She was usually pretty composed, so I knew that something serious was happening. I had been the family doctor for Judy and her husband, Bill, for about five years. I had delivered their son, Frank, a couple of years earlier. I knew her well. She asked if I would come to her parents' home before I went to the hospital that morning, the reason being that her father was very sick. I agreed without question; Judy wouldn't ask if it wasn't important.

I grabbed some toast on the way out of the house and followed the directions to Judy's parents' home. It was one of those $9,999.99 Florida specials from the 1950s near the railroad tracks. When I pulled up in front of the house, Judy and her mother were standing outside waiting. Judy was controlled. Mom was less composed; she was crying. Her hand shook visibly as she reached out to greet me. I went into the house, and there on the living room floor lay Judy's father, Delbert. He was semiconscious. That is, he would open his eyes and moan a little when I shook him. He had vomited a large amount of blood. The whole room reeked of the stench of vomitus and whiskey.

As I viewed this scene with the semiconscious man on the floor, the bloody vomit, and the smell of whiskey, I could feel my adrenaline rise a little. Why hadn't Judy told me that her father was an alcoholic, that he had reached the bottom of the bottle? That was certainly what it looked like. I got a little bit rude as I questioned Judy and her mother about Delbert's drinking habits. Both women were insistent that Delbert was not accustomed to drinking whiskey. They maintained that he had only taken some that morning in hopes that it would ease his stomach pain. I began to relent. Perhaps this wasn't a simple case of alcoholism. If what these two women were telling me was true, the whiskey may just have been the straw that broke the camel's back. He could have been bleeding in his stomach and been ready to vomit, drank some whiskey, and the whole mess came right back up and out onto the living room floor. As I listened to the story that Judy and her mother told me, I began to feel more than a little ashamed for being so quick to jump to conclusions.

In any case, there are times when you must put your feelings aside quickly and do something. Delbert's pulse was rapid and weak, his blood pressure was low. It looked like he had lost a lot of blood (but a pint of blood has a way of looking like a gallon when you spread it out on a living room floor). He needed treatment right away. He could die right there on the floor while I was debating about how much whiskey he had consumed or indulged my guilty feelings for jumping to the wrong conclusion.

First I called an ambulance. That done, I made a fast call to the hospital to arrange Delbert's admission. This was in the days when a doctor on a house call could hospitalize a patient without getting insurance forms filled out first. A four-bed ward cost about $50 a day. The ambulance arrived in a matter of minutes. Judy went with her father in the ambulance. I drove the five miles to the hospital in my own car while Judy's mother followed along in their vintage Ford. On the way to the hospital, I considered all the possible things that could be wrong with Delbert. Little did I know that this morbid, semiconscious man would show me something that would change my whole professional life.

The trip to the hospital took about 10 minutes. As soon as we got there, we put Delbert in a wheelchair. He seemed a little better, so we stopped by the x-ray department to get some pictures of his chest and abdomen. While we were in the x-ray department, the lab technician came over and started the blood tests. I loved working in this small, informal hospital. We could expedite matters like this and do the paperwork later. I fear those days are gone forever.

The x-rays showed that Delbert had black lung disease along with other spots on his lungs and some emphysema. He was a retired West Virginia coal miner, so we weren't surprised. The abdominal x-rays showed me nothing except that there was a rather large air bubble in his stomach. We took Delbert to his room and put him to bed. I started an IV while we waited for the first results of the blood tests. This case was going to be a challenge once we got Delbert "out of the woods." We really needed to know how all this started and why. That is one of the joys of being a doctor; you always get to search for "why." I had no idea what a long search this was going to be and of the impact that the answer would have on my life and the lives of untold numbers of other people.

The blood results began to come back in about 30 minutes. The blood loss had been sufficient to warrant a transfusion, so I ordered two pints of blood over the next 24 hours. I had learned not to go too fast in a case like this; the body needs a chance to adapt.

We used medications to quiet the stomach problems and began the search for the cause of Delbert's problem. Stomach x-rays with barium showed some active ulcers. Liver and brain scans showed cysts in both of these organs. After Delbert was stable, we did liver biopsies and found that the cysts contained a parasite named echinococcus. Blood tests then suggested that this parasitic infection probably involved the whole body—it was systemic. I felt safe in assuming that the cysts in the brain were from the same cause. There was a medication in the quinine family of drugs that we could use to treat this rare condition. Within about three weeks, Delbert's condition had improved enough so that I could send him home.

2

I'm Hooked and Don't Know It

About 10 days after Delbert went home, Judy called and told me that her dad had done "pretty well" for about a week, but then his feet began to hurt so bad that he was not able to stand up on them. I asked a few questions, and got very puzzled as she answered. Judy said that the skin on the bottoms of both her dad's feet was turning black, cracking and peeling off. It really hurt. I stopped by Delbert's house the next day to take a look. Sure enough, the bottoms of his feet were very dark, if not black. The skin was deeply cracked, and it looked like I could peel it off in large pieces with my fingernail. Where the dark, thick skin had already peeled off, it left very raw and painful areas. I had never seen anything like this before, nor have I since. It looked like some kind of armor plating.

Next began our long search for the answer. A dermatologist offered no help. Over a period of a few months we sent Delbert to three major medical centers in the southeastern United States. None of them were able to offer any insight into the problem with his feet. All three found out that he had black lung disease and emphysema. Two of them offered psychiatric diagnoses.

After all of this, Judy and her mother prevailed upon me to try just once more to find out what was wrong with Delbert and his feet. I had accepted the idea that doctors who were much smarter than I had not solved the problem, so how could they expect me to do it? Then I fell victim to flattery. Judy and her mother told me that I was the best doctor of them all. They pleaded with me to put Delbert back in the hospital just once more and try to find out what was wrong. If I couldn't find out, they would leave me alone. We would accept that there may be some things that simply are not knowable.

To make a long and technical story shorter, and perhaps a little less tedious, I exhausted my knowledge and ideas during the first couple of days of Delbert's hospital stay. I was stuck. Then I got a "last chance" idea. We had a new neuro (brain) surgeon on staff who had practiced general medicine about nine years before he studied surgery. He did his general surgery training for three years in the United States, after which he went to Japan to become a neurosurgeon. With this wide background I thought that perhaps he would have a fresh idea or two. I asked him to look Delbert over and let me know if he saw any possibilities that I might have overlooked.

After his examination and evaluation, Jim (the neurosurgeon) suggested that in Japan they talk about "dystrophy" as a cause for the kind of tissue changes we were seeing in Delbert's feet. Jim suggested that we do a myelogram up in the neck area, called a cervical myelogram. It is not without risk of complication. Jim's suggestion seemed to me to be based largely on intuition, but he finally convinced me that we might find our answer using this procedure.

I explained to Judy and her mother and father that Jim was suggesting a procedure that involved injecting a dye into the spinal canal down in the low-back region. The x-ray table is then tipped so that the head goes lower than the feet, causing the dye to run into the neck and head. X-rays are then taken of the dye after it has moved up the spinal canal into the neck region. I explained that the dye could cause a reaction and be somewhat risky. I also explained that I wasn't quite sure what we would get from this study, but that Jim was somewhat optimistic, and I didn't have any better suggestions. They enthusiastically supported the procedure. We did the cervical myelogram. Lo and behold, there on the outside surface of the meningeal membrane (dura mater) that covers the spinal cord, about halfway down the neck on the back (posterior) side, was a plaque of calcium about the size of a dime. Jim was jubilant. I was awed by his genius. Delbert, Judy and her mom were seeing the first ray of hope in several months.

Now came the soul-searching. Delbert had gone through the diagnostic test (cervical myelogram) with no problem. But now we were thinking about doing a very serious operation. It could be life-threatening or cause paralysis from the neck down. The potential benefit was to clear up a skin condition on this man's feet. We weren't at all sure that the operation would help his feet.

Jim was pushing to surgically remove the plaque. He was a surgeon; surgeons cut things out. But, to his credit, I had to keep in mind that he had found this plaque that no one else had even suspected.

Delbert, his wife and his daughter were pushing for the surgery. They saw it as doing something with some chance of success. This was better then doing nothing, which seemed to offer no chance of improvement. Delbert said he would rather die than have his feet remain this way. I asked how he would feel about it if he was paralyzed. He let me know that he would also rather die than be paralyzed. He told me not to worry; he would see to things should paralysis result—he had a point. But how do you not worry about such things? It was a question of his right to take a calculated risk in order to improve the quality of his own life. All my training said the risk was unwarranted. The risk-benefit ratio was an atrocity. But whose life was it anyway? Who was I to play God to this poor, suffering man? After much agonizing and soul-searching, I agreed, and we scheduled the surgery.

Jim would do the operation, and I would be the assistant. In real terms this agreement meant that, for a few hours of my life, I would do everything that Jim told me to do in exactly the way that he told me to do it.

3

A Glimpse Of The Core

On the morning of surgery I was still feeling concerned about whether or not I had made the right decision. Soon it would be too late to change my mind. On the one hand, when it was over Delbert could be cured. On the other hand, he could be paralyzed, or he could get meningitis...or he could die. But if the calcium plaque was allowed to remain, it might grow and have to be removed later. Its presence could cause paralysis later on...maybe. There just wasn't a clear answer in Delbert's case as far as I could see.

Jim and I met in the doctor's lounge. We exchanged niceties, got into our surgical gowns, and then went into the operating room to oversee the positioning of our patient for surgery. Delbert was placed in a sitting position, strapped into an anesthesia chair with his head bent forward somewhat so that the back of his neck was stretched out and exposed. In this position he was put to sleep. The heart monitor was in place and working. He was breathing through a ventilation system that showed each breath and the size of it. All you had to do was watch and you could see how he was doing.

Jim and I went out to the sinks to scrub up. I kept my concerns about whether the surgery was warranted to myself; after all, there was nothing to gain now by expressing my doubts about the efficacy of what we were about to do. Once we were scrubbed (and, ideally, sterile from the fingertips and fingernails to the elbows), we went into the operating room where we were gowned and gloved. Zero hour was upon us.

We scrubbed the operation site with a sterilizing solution that turned it all reddish brown. Then we hung the green drapes around the operative site and taped them into position on Delbert's neck. Delbert was no longer a man. He was now only a reddish-brown patch of skin about two inches wide and four to five inches long. Instinctively my personal compassion for him was put aside. When you are doing surgery you have to subordinate your feelings about cutting and mutilating a fellow human being. You have to detach. Focusing on the operative site, which has been made impersonal by taking it out of the context of the total person, helps you do this. It did. Now I was a surgical first assistant. If Jim wanted me to stand on my head while brushing my teeth and singing "The Star-Spangled Banner," I would give it my best shot.

Jim made a vertical incision right down the middle of the back of Delbert's neck. I always marvel at how well a good surgeon can use exactly enough pressure with the scalpel to cut just through the skin without damaging the deeper tissues. I used the electrocautery to stop the bleeding from a few small blood vessels in the skin. This cautery machine buzzes and gives you the acrid smell of burning flesh when you touch the end of it to the patient. On the second cut, Jim went through the ligaments on the back of the neck. After I cauterized a few more blood vessels, we began the laborious task of separating the very tough ligaments from the bony surfaces of the spinal column in the back of the neck. As Jim did this work, I used instruments called retractors that hook around body tissue and allowed me to pull it out of his way.

Next we had to remove the back parts of two of the bony vertebrae in the middle of the neck so that we could get to the calcium plaque on the membrane inside the spinal canal. This membrane is totally surrounded by bone.

All the vertebrae of your spine are shaped so that they form a canal that goes all the way from the base of your skull to just a couple of inches above your tailbone. In front of the canal is the supporting part of the vertebra that is called the body (vertebral body). The bodies are the supporting parts of your spine. Your spinal column is a pile or stack of these vertebral bodies with softer shock absorber discs interposed between each two of the vertebral bodies. In addition to their function as shock absorbers, the discs allow for bending and rotation movements of the spine. Just behind the stack of vertebral bodies and discs that support your body is the spinal canal. This canal offers protective housing for the spinal cord as it extends from your head to your tail.

Inside this spinal canal is a membrane system that further houses and protects the spinal cord. This membrane system also carries blood vessels that nurture the spinal cord and its nerve roots. The membrane system is three-layered: the outermost layer is called the dura mater; the middle layer is called the arachnoid membrane; and the innermost layer is called the pia mater. The inside layer adheres snugly to the spinal cord. There is a fluid between all other layers. This fluid lubricates so that one membrane can glide in relationship to another and the spine can move about in acts of bending and twisting. The fluid, called cerebrospinal fluid, also carries nutrients and takes away waste products.

This membrane system is officially called the meninges. When it gets infected or inflamed, it hurts like you can't imagine, and causes what is called meningitis. It can be a deadly and/or very crippling disease.

The outermost layer of the membrane system, the dura mater, is tough and waterproof. It protects everything inside of it. It totally encloses the brain and spinal cord. It was on the outer surface of this dura mater membrane that our dime-sized calcium plaque was located. Since the plaque was on the outer surface of the meningeal membrane system, our plan was to remove it without nicking or cutting any of the membrane. To do so would be to open an avenue for infection that could result in meningitis. It was decided that Jim would very carefully scrape off the calcium plaque while I held this section of membrane perfectly still. If I did my job properly, he would not have an accident and cut the membrane.

After we had removed the backsides of these cervical vertebrae, there it was in all its glistening glory—the dura mater membrane. And there was our calcium plaque looking at us from right in the center of the operative field. The nurse now took over my job and held the muscles to the side, while I took a pair of forceps in each hand. Now all I had to do was hold this dura mater membrane perfectly still for Jim as he very carefully removed the calcium plaque. Everything was going well until I tried to stop the movement of the dura mater membrane. It wouldn't hold still no matter what I did. It kept moving toward and away from us rather slowly, yet rhythmically and irresistibly. I don't recall the exact conversation that Jim and I had, but it was full of comments about my inability to perform a simple task. My responses cast a few aspersions upon anyone who thought this was such a simple task. My pride was hurt. I was embarrassed at my own ineptitude. But I also became very curious about this strange phenomenon that I was witnessing. Ultimately, Jim removed the plaque without a slip of his knife, in spite of the irrepressible moving membrane. I discovered that this rhythmically moving membrane's performance to which I was so intimately connected was new to everyone else in the operating room. It was not synchronous with Delbert's breathing. That fact was clearly

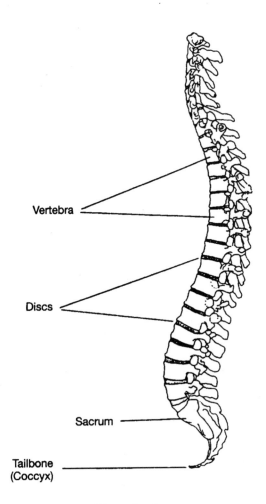

Vertebra

Discs

Sacrum

Tailbone
(Coccyx)

Illustration 1
Side view of spinal column showing vertebra and discs

seen on the breathing machine. It did not synchronize with the heart rate (pulse) that I could see on the cardiac monitor. It was another bodily rhythm that, at about 10 cycles per minute, seemed very reliable and consistent. I had never seen nor read about this rhythm, nor had the neurosurgeon, the anesthesiologist, the nurses or the intern. Little did I know we were looking at the "core" of Delbert.

4

I'm Hooked and I Know It

Since I met Delbert that first day, as he was lying on the floor of his living room in blood and vomit, my life began to change. First he made me understand that I shouldn't jump to conclusions. Then he let me feel guilty for a while because I had jumped to the conclusion that his was a case of alcoholism. Next he introduced me to a rare parasitic infection and showed me what it could do to a human being. I had never seen liver and brain cysts from a parasitic infection before. Delbert then showed me that big medical centers and professors/doctors don't necessarily know everything. They didn't figure out what Jim's intuition had told him. I began learning about the conflict between rational and analytic thought versus hunches and intuition. I had agonized a great deal about whether or not to approve the cervical myelogram procedure and then the surgery. Delbert showed me that it was his choice, not mine. The risk-benefit ratio was his to evaluate. I could recommend, but I couldn't and shouldn't tell him what to do. Delbert taught me to respect his rights as a human being.

Then, at surgery, Delbert afforded me my first look at what was to become the craniosacral system. He did it in such a way that my pride was injured. I was embarrassed at my own inability to hold a membrane still. He also stirred a curiosity in me that would not be quieted. Partially because of the pride and embarrassment, and partially because of my own curiosity, I would not forget the vision of that small area of dura mater membrane moving continually toward and away from us as I tried hard to hold it still. He made it a memorable experience. Wonder of wonders, I was experiencing the privilege of seeing firsthand the physiological performance of an as-yet-undiscovered bodily system. It would turn out to be another system, just like the cardiovascular system, the digestive system and the like.

Delbert wanted to be sure I didn't escape, so he healed his feet in a few months and was fine. I certainly didn't understand the implications of moving membranes and healing feet, but I would find out. As it turned out, I only had to wait a matter of months until I saw an advertisement in an osteopathic journal for a five-day seminar in cranial osteopathy. I vaguely knew that these were the people who manipulated the bones of the skull. At that time I was of the belief that once an adult, your skull bones are all fused together and can't move. Your skull is solid like a coconut.

I swallowed my disbelief and attended the seminar on cranial osteopathy. I felt the bone movement with my hands immediately and knew that the movement I felt was somehow linked to the irrepressible moving membrane that caused me so much embarrassment during Delbert's surgery.

Delbert had done a good job. I was hooked and I knew it. Thank you, Delbert.

Incidentally, Delbert moved to Texas after a while and I lost track of him. I then heard about 10 years later that he died of lung cancer.

He certainly did a good job on me.

5

The Craniosacral System

After some years of research, we now know that each of us has a craniosacral system inside that is rhythmically moving all the days we are alive. We have learned to monitor this craniosacral rhythm with our hands upon almost any part of a human body. Just as we are able to make certain inferences from heart rhythm and breathing activity about the cardiovascular and respiratory systems, we are now able to gather information about the condition and function of the craniosacral rhythm in and on various regions and parts of the human body.

When certain body parts or regions do not move rhythmically in response to the gentle urging of the craniosacral system, we are able to localize areas of trouble in the body. We don't necessarily know what the trouble is, but we know where it is, and that is a powerful start in problem solving.

The craniosacral system itself is made up of: (1) the three-layered membrane system that we call the meninges; (2) the cerebrospinal fluid which is enclosed by this membrane system; and (3) the structures within the membrane system that control fluid input and outflow for the system. What I have just described is a semi-closed hydraulic system that uses the waterproof dura mater membrane (the outer layer of the three-layered membrane system) as its fluid enclosure barrier. It uses cerebrospinal fluid as the hydraulic component of the system. It uses the choroid system within the brain ventricles as the fluid input component, and it uses the arachnoid system as its fluid outflow component.

The powerful influence that the craniosacral system exercises upon total body function happens in large part because the system encloses the brain and spinal cord as well as the pituitary and pineal glands. Since the brain and spinal cord are more or less masters of your total nervous system, it is easy to see that the craniosacral system, by means of its effect upon the environment of the brain and spinal cord, has powerful influence over a wide variety of bodily functions. And via its influence upon the pituitary (master) gland and the pineal gland, the craniosacral system has a powerful effect upon the function of your endocrine system and the hormones that it secretes.

The membranous fluid barrier (dura mater) of the craniosacral system attaches to the bones of the skull on the inside. This dura mater membrane is actually the lining of the skull. We have shown through our research at Michigan State University that the skull bones must be in continual, minute motion in order to accommodate the constant fluid pressure changes that are going on within the membrane boundary of the semi-closed hydraulic system. When skull bones lose their ability to move in response to the changing pressures of the craniosacral system, the function of this system becomes compromised and symptoms may occur.

As CranioSacral Therapists we know about the attachments of the dura mater membranes to the skull bones, to the vertebrae of the upper neck, to the sacrum in the low back, and to all the little openings in the skull and vertebral column that allow passage for major nerves going to all parts of the body. We know how to find the areas of restricted movement that compromise craniosacral system function. And we know how to re-establish normal accommodation motion in all of these areas. In doing this work we are often able to improve the function of the nervous and endocrine systems by improving the environment in which these systems do their work.

6

Early Experiences With CranioSacral Therapy

My initial work with CranioSacral Therapy as a treatment method began with a few headache patients who responded very well. One case was rather intriguing. He was the first severe-headache patient with whom I tried using these techniques. The patient was in the U.S. Navy during World War II. He was standing in the vicinity of a large gun/cannon on his ship when the cannon was fired. He had neglected to put in his ear plugs or wear his ear muffs. His headache began immediately and was accompanied by a loud noise in his ears. The pain and noise were unrelenting. He underwent every kind of treatment the U.S. Navy could think of, but found no relief. Finally the Navy gave him a medical discharge with a disability allowance. He had been suffering this pain for about 25 years. How he happened to come to my office, I do not know. I evaluated his craniosacral system and found the skull bones on the left side of his head to be jammed inward and stuck. There was no movement in these bones. I was very lucky, and successfully released this "stuckness." The left side of his head expanded immediately. As this expansion and release of stuckness occurred, he became exuberant. His head pain left him right there as I worked on him. His ear noise took a few weeks to stop. I only saw the man three times. His pain of more than 25 years' duration was gone after the first treatment. As far as I know, it never came back. I'm sure he would have contacted me again if it had reoccurred.

After this experience with the Navy veteran's headache, I began working with many headache patients. Most of them had suffered for many years and had undergone a wide variety of treatment programs. I learned a lot about headaches and the efficacy of CranioSacral Therapy as an approach to the chronic, severe and often partially disabled headache patient. Since the beginning, my experience shows that about 80 to 85 percent of resistant long-term headache patients respond favorably to CranioSacral Therapy. The really good part is that, in the majority of these successfully treated people, once the problem is solved, it stays solved. The patient is not dependent upon a lifetime of periodic CranioSacral Therapy sessions. (The therapy feels so good, though, that many of them want more even after the headaches are gone.)

In order to set the hook deeper in me, another patient came along. This was a 16-year-old "retarded" boy. His mother insisted, in a very nice way, that I try this new treatment method, CranioSacral Therapy, on her son. Russell, the son's name, had contracted meningitis as an infant. The meningitis was supposedly responsible for his ongoing mental retardation. I had no previous experience using CranioSacral Therapy with this type of problem. I had no idea that there could be any improvement. However, at the gentle and irresistible urging of Russell's mother, I decided we could try.

Russell's uncle was a prominent surgeon. He had seen to it that Russell received every kind of conventional medical treatment that was available through the years since his meningitis. I was quite dubious, but nonetheless I sent Russell for an electroencephalogram (EEG) just to see what we might find. Jim, the neurosurgeon who was present during my introduction to the craniosacral system, interpreted the EEG for

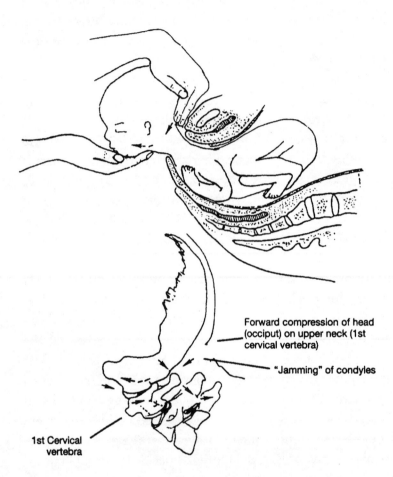

Forward compression of head
(occiput) on upper neck (1st
cervical vertebra)

"Jamming" of condyles

1st Cervical
vertebra

Illustration 2
Jamming of occiput (skull) into upper neck
(cervical) vertebra and how it can happen

me. The thought that stayed in my mind from the EEG inter-pretation was that there seemed to be some brain tissue irritation, probably due to reduced blood supply from the arteries on the underside of the brain. This might explain how meningitis could result in "retardation." The membranes involved in the previous meningitis might still be swollen and/or have adhesions that partially obstructed the arteries that supply blood to Russell's brain. If the drainage veins were also partly obstructed, they could easily produce a back pres-sure. This might result in a stagnation of blood in the brain. These conditions would make it difficult for fresh blood to get where it was needed.

I decided that I would focus treatment on improving the drainage of oxygen-poor (venous) blood from the brain and upon improving the supply of oxygen-rich (arterial) blood to the brain. I had these bony handles (skull bones) on the dura mater membrane system that I could use to change abnormal membrane tension within the skull vault and the spinal canal. If I could reduce abnormal tension, I might have a chance at loosening any adhesions. Between the tension reduction and the adhesion loosening, we might get better blood drainage and an improvement in fresh blood supply to Russell's brain. Initially I used some medications to improve blood supply, but I focused mostly on CranioSacral Therapy. I improvised methods that would enable me to use the bones of the skull, the upper neck and the low back in order to get the dura mater membrane and the other meningeal membranes moving. I saw Russell for treatment twice weekly. Within three weeks, Russell's mother reported that he no longer took afternoon naps. He just wasn't as tired and sleepy as usual. In about four months, Russell's academic tutor reported that he was doing well and suggested that her services be discontinued. Russell then mainstreamed into the 10th grade.

I continued to treat Russell with CranioSacral Therapy on a weekly basis for about a year. Ultimately, Russell graduated from high school without difficulty, attended and graduated from a junior college, and now, about 20 years later, manages the pickup and delivery services for a large medical laboratory. He supervises approximately 20 drivers, owns and operates some rental properties, and lives independently in his own home in another town away from his family. Russell was evaluated by a psychologist before I began his treatment and again a year later. In summary, his estimated IQ went up about 20 points. This kind of successful treatment experience really hooks you. CranioSacral Therapy had me, and I hadn't even named it yet.

I had worked with Russell's case before I accepted the faculty position at Michigan State University. This experience let me know how CranioSacral Therapy might influence brain function. After Russell, while still in private practice, I had experienced some success with hyperactive and learning-disabled children. Once installed as a clinician-researcher at Michigan State University, I began work with children who were having trouble in school. The majority of these children were either hyperactive or dyslexic.

Our early success in the clinic with hyperactive children was most encouraging. The hyperactive child would often fall asleep on the treatment table after we made the craniosacral system correction. Usually this problem was found at the base of the skull in the back where the head joins the neck.

There was usually a jamming forward of the head on the neck and then an extreme tightness of the neck muscles that maintained this malposition. Once we released that bony "stuckness," the dura mater membrane system loosened and the hyperactive child began to behave more normally. Frequently, dietary restrictions could then be relaxed. Food allergies significantly improved. At that time the Feingold diet was being widely used to control hyperactive behavior. This diet eliminated sugar, food coloring, etc., and was difficult to follow. CranioSacral Therapy eased this difficult situation significantly. If we did not find the jamming of the skull (occipital bone) forward on the neck, we observed that the hyperactivity was probably due to some other cause. Frequently there were psychological reasons for the hyperactive behavior when the craniosacral system was not at fault.

I say "we" because, by this time, I began to have a constant and generous supply of graduate students working with me. They were learning CranioSacral Therapy quite easily. It was very encouraging to see how easily these techniques could be taught.

I theorized that when the hyperactivity was due to craniosacral system dysfunction, the problem may have occurred during the birth process. Quite often the baby's head is bent backwards excessively (hyperextended) in an attempt to speed the delivery after the infant's head is partially out of the mother's birth canal. Persistence of this hyperextension could be the culprit. I feel very strongly that if this condition could be diagnosed and corrected in the first few days of life, a significant reduction (probably 50 percent) of the hyperactive-child problem could be alleviated. Our success rate was nearly 100 percent when the hyperactive child presented the jammed condition of the head forward on the neck. About 50 percent of the hyperactive children we saw in our clinic had this condition. The other 50 percent were hyperactive for other reasons.

The clinic in those early years at Michigan State University also attracted large numbers of dyslexic children. We found that many dyslexic children presented with a craniosacral system problem that was located in the right side of the head

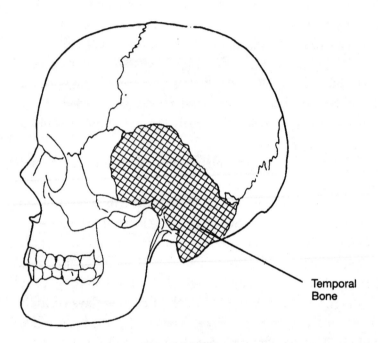

Temporal
Bone

Illustration 3
Temporal bone location in skull

involving the ear and the mastoid region. Actually, the key problem turned out to be the right temporal bone and its attached dura mater membranes. Once this condition was corrected and craniosacral system function was returned to normal, the reading problems disappeared in a very high percentage (about 70 percent) of these children. I remember, as though it was yesterday, one 16-year-old boy whose special education teacher brought him to our clinic from about 100 miles away. The teacher said that the boy (Mike) was reading on a fourth-grade level at the very best. He was assigned to a special classroom. Mike was beginning to show self-destructive behavior due to low self-esteem. He was about a 200-pound, six-foot-tall boy whom I didn't want mad at me.

During our first treatment session I found and corrected by about 80 percent the right temporal bone and related dura mater membrane problem. Due to the distance traveled, it was agreed that Mike would return in two weeks. Our usual routine was to treat the child once a week. I saw him the second time and completed the craniosacral system correction of the right side of his head. Mike said very little. His teacher said that there was some improvement in both reading skill and attitude. He would return in two weeks. I felt that the craniosacral system correction was complete.

In two weeks' time Mike returned. This time both he and his teacher were smiling and very happy. Mike was reading out of 10th-grade books without difficulty. I asked Mike what had happened. He said that he could see two or three words at a time. Before, he had to see each letter in the word individually, memorize the letter sequence, and then try to think of the word from his recall of the letter sequence. He was very happy, as was his kind and caring teacher. Four weeks had lapsed since Mike had undergone his first CranioSacral Therapy session. In three sessions of about 20 minutes each, an hour in treatment time all together, he had progressed from a self-destructive, learning-disabled, fourth-grade-level reader to a happy 10th-grade-level student. Boy, was I hooked.

The children's clinic continued, and the variety of problems widened. We began to get reports that constipation problems with these children were improving. Attitudes and levels of displayed affection were improving. Then we began to hear from parents that some of the children who also suffered seizures were not having the seizure episodes anymore. The big question was: Could we reduce seizure medication? We tried slowly and cautiously, and it worked about half the time. Some children were actually able to discontinue their medication entirely without seizures. The majority of these children, however, were able to remain seizure-free by taking about one-half or less of their previous anticonvulsant medication dosage.

7

The Horizons Broaden

If I wasn't totally hooked on CranioSacral Therapy by now, the next experience did it. I went to France and England to teach in 1978. The osteopaths over there wanted to learn CranioSacral Therapy and arranged for me to give some five-day seminars on the system and its therapeutic uses. As I was preparing for the seminar in the city of Nice, in the south of France, an enrollee from Brussels, Belgium, asked me if I would treat a little 2 1/2-year-old boy as a demonstration model during the five days of the seminar. That meant that, at the end of each class day, I would perform the CranioSacral Therapy techniques we had learned that day on the little boy. The boy, Olivier is his name, was a victim of some problem that had occurred during or shortly after his obstetrical delivery. He was labeled as having cerebral palsy. He wore thick glasses. His eyes were crossed. He was spastic and paralyzed on the right side of his body. Both his right arm and right leg were essentially useless to him. He could not chew effectively and had some difficulty with his swallowing. All of his food was run through a blender and fed to him by an adult. I had never treated a child like this before and did not have much hope of helping him.

On the third day of the seminar the techniques I used were focused on the correction of improper dura mater membrane tensions in the forehead and extending back about three-fourths of the way inside the head. In order to accomplish this release of dura mater membrane tension, I had to free the frontal bone, which is the bone of the forehead. I could then effectively use this bone as the handle on the dura mater membrane inside the skull to stretch that membrane.

In order to do this I simply lifted the forehead toward the ceiling ever so gently with the patient lying comfortably on his back. His face was looking straight up. I began my gentle lift aimed at freeing the frontal bone (forehead bone) from the parietal bones. The parietal bones form the top of the head just behind the frontal. I had previously felt a ridge on the left side of Olivier's head where the frontal bone was over-lapping the parietal bone. In my experience thus far this overlap had been a rare finding. It happens often in infants, but nature usually straightens it out during the first year of life. As I continued to gently lift Olivier's frontal bone, there was an audible noise as the bony overlapping corrected itself. The way this happened reminded me that, when dealing with a human body, a small force over a long time can do more than a strong force over a short time. This is because the small force recruits much less resistance from the patient's body. I had been holding the frontal bone up for about five minutes when the overlapping of the two bones of Olivier's skull corrected.

The next day at 4:00 p.m. when Olivier came to class to be the demonstration model, there was a very loud commotion. I could not see what was going on, and I did not understand French, so I didn't know what all the shouting, clapping and cheering was about. Soon I knew. Olivier was holding onto his mother's hand and was walking into the lecture hall. He had never walked before. I was astonished, but tried to be cool as a good professor should. Olivier's mother was crying and laughing at the same time. Soon she was kiss-

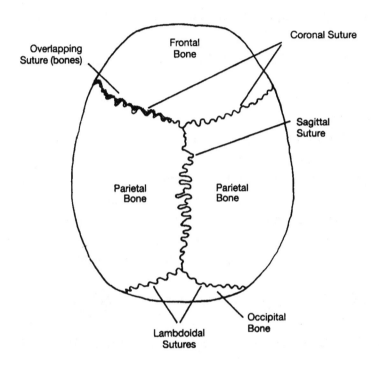

Illustration 4
Top view of skull showing sutures and location
of Olivier's overlap between frontal and
left parietal bones

ing my hands and generally embarrassing me with this unbridled display of emotion. It seems that at 4:00 a.m. Olivier awakened, called his mother into his bedroom, and informed her that he could walk. He said that the mean man in his body that wouldn't let him walk before was gone. Within 12 hours, Olivier learned to walk so that he could enter the classroom that day holding his mother's hand and walking together with her for the first time.

Olivier and his mother followed me from France to England and then back to Michigan, where they remained for three months. During this time I treated Olivier with CranioSacral Therapy about twice a week. By the time we finished he was walking rather well. He did drag his right foot a little, but he wasn't spastic at all. He was cutting his food, feeding himself, and chewing and swallowing on his own at all meals. He no longer wore glasses, and he wasn't cross-eyed anymore. He was bright and possessed a remarkably good sense of humor.

I did not see Olivier again for almost 12 years. In August 1990, his mother called from Brussels and said that Olivier wanted to meet me because I had been the one who allowed him to walk. What a thrill to see this 15-year-old boy who walked with a limp but did most everything else rather well.

The hook of CranioSacral Therapy was now inexorably set deeply inside of me. It began with Delbert, and now I knew that CranioSacral Therapy was no longer just a subject for research. It was more, much more.

Following my experience with Olivier there came a stream of spastic, paralyzed children. Many of them improved a great deal. Olivier is the one who is so deeply branded in my memory.

8

Other Uses for CranioSacral Therapy

So now I knew that CranioSacral Therapy was capable of producing excellent results in slow, hyperactive, dyslexic, and spastic cerebral-palsied children. Next came autistic children and newborns. I received a research grant to work with autistic children over a three-year period. At the time when the grant ended, we were making some very significant progress at a center for autism. The children were inflicting much less pain on themselves, displaying affection toward other human beings, and showing greatly improved social behavior.

Unfortunately, the research money for this study dried up. I don't know how far we might have gone. There was a regression in the autistic children when they were not treated with CranioSacral Therapy for three or four months. It was clear that we needed to go further with our work. We did have a few private-patient autistic children come to our clinic at the University. One of them was 6 years old and had only begun to display autistic behavior about 1 1/2 years earlier. I'm sure the diagnosis was valid because it was made at the Bethesda Naval Hospital and confirmed at the University of Virginia Medical School. The father was discharged from the Navy on hardship because of the child. We treated the boy about six times immediately upon his arrival in Michigan. His improvement was so marked that the state evaluation team in Michigan did not label him autistic. He was called developmentally slow. They put him in a regular classroom and he did fine. I know that we have a lot more work in the field of autism that could be done by well-trained CranioSacral Therapists. We did learn something about the differentiation of autism from childhood schizophrenia by the evaluation of the craniosacral system.

We did a blind study with children who had been rated on the Rimland Developmental Landmark Scale. This scale diagnoses both autism and schizophrenia. I made my own diagnosis, based on the craniosacral system characteristics, on 63 children who had been rated by Dr. Rimland. I did not know his results before I gave my own impression. The agreement between Dr. Rimland's diagnosis, based on developmental landmarks, and my own diagnosis, based on craniosacral system evaluation, was very high. It was extremely improbable that this agreement could have been reached by chance.

Lest you get the impression that I was spending all of my life treating brain-dysfunctioning children, I would like to tell you about some of the uses for CranioSacral Therapy we found that did not involve dysfunctional children.

We found that CranioSacral Therapy may shorten and ease the discomfort of obstetrical labor for both mother and child. I was teaching in England at the European School of Osteopathy in Maidstone, Kent, during the fall of 1977. One of the student's wives had been in labor for three days. The doctors had scheduled her for Caesarean section delivery that afternoon. The student, Simon, was quite upset about the possibility of Caesarean rather than vaginal delivery of their first child. But the labor was long, it was not progressing, and his wife Deborah's blood pressure was getting dangerously high. The surgery was to be done in about four hours. Simon and I had never met before. He was trying to effectively divide his time between the hospital and my seminar. He came up after my first morning lecture and asked if there was anything I could recommend within the realm of CranioSacral Therapy that might be helpful. My conventional medical background was not far behind me, and I was concerned about the non-productive labor and the high blood pressure. I advised Simon to allow the scheduled Caesarean section to be performed. However he had four hours during which he could try a CranioSacral Therapy technique that might, we hoped, affect the pituitary gland positively and cause the stalled labor to effectively recommence. I also showed him CranioSacral techniques that could lower blood pressure. Simon left all excited and ready to try. He was back within three hours.

Deborah had gone into strong, effective labor while Simon was applying the CranioSacral Therapy technique. She delivered a healthy girl named Hannah within 30 minutes of the time Simon began to work on her craniosacral system. He did not even get to the blood pressure techniques because Deborah delivered the baby and her blood pressure came down naturally. The doctors were baffled—but happy. Simon never told them what he did. We visit with Simon, Deborah, Hannah and their youngest daughter, Charlotte, almost annually when we are in Europe or when they come to the States. We are good friends. Hannah has often heard all about what CranioSacral Therapy did for her. Incidentally, I treated Hannah on the fourth day of her life as a demonstration before the class in Maidstone. She was born into instant fame.

Since that time, CranioSacral Therapy has proven to be very helpful and efficacious for mothers during pregnancy, delivery and postpartum (after delivery). The treated mother's incidence of back problems and postpartum blues seems much less than for those who do not receive CranioSacral Therapy.

We also like to treat well babies with CranioSacral Therapy. Dr. MacDonald, my colleague at The Upledger Institute in Palm Beach County, Florida, did CranioSacral Therapy on all newborn infants at the hospital where he was on staff in Maine. He did this over a period of five-plus years. All infants were treated at least once before they left the hospital to go home. During the first year of life the incidence of illness requiring hospitalization for the infants treated with CranioSacral Therapy was less than half the incidence of hospitalizations for infants born at a neighboring hospital where they did not receive CranioSacral Therapy.

Just a few months ago, a good friend and patient was telling me that their new baby, about six weeks old, was crying and colicky every night. Both mother and father were suffering from sleep deprivation. The pediatrician didn't have the answer. I suggested that they bring their new daughter in to see me. The crying child fell asleep during the first Cranio-Sacral Therapy session and slept all the way back to Miami. She slept for almost 10 hours. Three treatments were all that was required to completely end the problem. The craniosacral problem was an abnormally high tension in the dura mater membrane. This high tension was stemming from a twisted pelvis that probably occurred during delivery and remained stuck in the twisted position. This abnormal pelvic twist put tension into the dura mater membrane within the spinal canal. The tension was transmitted to the upper neck and head by the dura mater membrane system. The vagus nerve, which powerfully affects both stomach and bowel function (as well as having a big influence on heart rhythm and breathing), passes out of the base of the skull in a position that can easily be compromised by abnormal dura mater membrane tension. The craniosacral evaluation revealed the problem, and it was very easy to correct. The child is fine now.

CranioSacral Therapy is an excellent modality to use for a wide variety of infant distress problems such as colic, asthma, floppy baby syndrome and so on. The floppy baby is the one who is just like a rag doll. Most of the time the pediatricians don't know what causes this problem or what to do about it. Quite often a single CranioSacral Therapy session is all that is required to correct the problem. The dura mater membrane system is usually under very high and abnormal tension. The CranioSacral Therapist must find the reason for the abnormal tension and correct it if possible. If the problem is uncorrectable, there is usually some CranioSacral technique that will give temporary relief. We are most happy to teach parents or guardians how to do these techniques when ongoing treatment is required. They can then treat their child daily themselves and thus have a degree of independence from us, while gaining benefit for their child.

Recently, while I was conducting an advanced Cranio-Sacral Therapy seminar in Bordeaux, France, a student presented a case of a floppy baby with a diagnosis of neurological damage due to oxygen deprivation at birth. I treated this child with CranioSacral Therapy. As the dura mater membrane system relaxed, you could literally see this four-month-old child begin to move its arms and legs, control its head, neck and torso, and give out a robust cry rather than a whimper. Within about 30 minutes from the time the treatment began, the child appeared normal. We do a lot of very good work with infants and toddlers. It is my feeling that a craniosacral evaluation and treatment program during the first months of life could reduce the brain dysfunctions of children by at least 50 percent.

What kind of adult problems does CranioSacral Therapy deal with? The spectrum of efficacy with adult problems (and for adults without problems) is almost inestimable. Earlier in this writing I referred to my first glimpse of the craniosacral system in action during Delbert's surgery as a glimpse of the "core." I really believe this is true. I'm not quite sure as yet what the core is all about, but I do know that at times the craniosacral system feels like the entrée into the deepest region of the patient's (and my own) total being. I'm not quite sure as yet what the "total being" is all about, but it feels like the craniosacral system is where it all comes together, whatever it is.

Consequently, there are a lot of very well and together adults who want and receive CranioSacral Therapy on a regular basis. Usually about once a month is what they would like. Because of demand that is disproportionate to supply, what they can get may be much less. My own practice at The Upledger Institute is composed of about 50 percent healthcare professionals of one kind or another from all over the North American continent and Europe. This says to me that CranioSacral Therapy must provide these people significant benefit, otherwise they wouldn't travel so far to receive treatment. Most of these healthcare professionals come for a week, which amounts to four or five consecutive treatments about once a year. They tell me how much better they feel not only physically, but also emotionally and spiritually. It is as though this craniosacral system is a "core" system where the control mechanisms of body, mind, emotion and spirit all come together.

From a subjective point of view, well persons who receive CranioSacral Therapy claim to have more energy and feel happier and more contented. They contract fewer infections and are sick less severely and for shorter periods of time than before they received CranioSacral Therapy. From my point of view, it would seem that the function of the immune system is enhanced, stress levels are reduced, hormonal balance is improved, and a sense of well-being is heightened.

Many healthcare professionals first discovered the benefits of CranioSacral Therapy by observing their patients. Most of the healthcare professionals whom I treat are developing the expertise necessary to do CranioSacral Therapy themselves. Some, however, have only seen what other therapists have been able to accomplish with this work. In any case, we treat lots of relatively well people who have either seen the positive effects of CranioSacral Therapy on their patients, or have received the treatment initially for a complaint and wanted to continue out of the negative complaint zone, through the neutral zone, and into the enhancement of the total being zone. This is a new concept for a disease-oriented society. Usually we assume that we are fine until we get sick. Cranio-Sacral Therapy can increase your well-being assets so that you don't have to get sick. More about the core aspects of the craniosacral system a little later.

As you may recall, headache was one category of problem that I first learned to treat using CranioSacral Therapy. Since that beginning about 20 years ago, I have successfully treated thousands of headache patients. The success rate is, I'm sure, well above 80 percent, no matter what the cause. We do of course encounter psychoemotional reasons for headaches in many cases. Craniosacral evaluation and treatment techniques are very helpful in identifying and treating the headache that is a symptom of deep psycho-emotional problems. More about headaches as we discuss SomatoEmotional Release and Therapeutic Imagery and Dialogue.

9

A Treatment for Depression

CranioSacral Therapy also produces excellent results in what is called endogenous depression. This is the "depression for no reason." Things just seem totally futile. There is no manic mood swing, you just stay down in the dumps. We have found that this type of depression frequently has a craniosacral system cause. There is a compression in three places. It is such a consistent finding that we have named it the Compression/Depression Triad.

The compressions are located in the floor of the skull vault in the center, halfway between the two temples. This is where two key bones of the skull vault floor meet. If they have been jammed together by a blow on the forehead or on the back of the head and have not released, this jamming and "stuckness" (or compression as we call it) may, over time, produce a similar jamming or compression at the base of the skull onto the neck and at the base of the lumbar spine onto the sacrum. I have also seen the compression at the lower end of the spine cause the other two compressions. This usually happens as a result of a fall on your derrière. As yet I have not (to my knowledge) seen the head-neck compression cause the other two compressions. When one causes the other two, it may take months or even years for the compression triad to come to completion and cause the psychoemotional depressive state.

When this compression triad is the cause of the depression, the mood will often lift as you obtain the therapeutic release of the compressions.

Just last week I found a compression triad in a 53-year-old lady who had been suffering from depression for about six years. She stated that she had also been depressed when she was in her early 20s. That previous depression had responded to psychotherapy. She said that this bout of depression felt different somehow. She couldn't "shake it," and psychotherapy did not seem to help.

She came to me because she was suffering from sciatic pain in her right leg. The pain had been rather constant for several months. She had gotten no help from the family doctor, the orthopedist or the neurosurgeon. Craniosacral evaluation revealed excessive dura mater membrane tension coming from the pelvis and base of the spine. The lower part of the compression triad was present. Craniosacral system evaluation in the head showed the other two compression components to be present. I successfully released the two head-end compressions and got started on the lower end of the craniosacral system during the first appointment. I saw her a week later. As I successfully released the compression at the base of the spine, she spontaneously laughed a little and told me that the weight of the world had just lifted from her shoulders, and that a big lead weight came off her chest. She then remembered a fall on her rear end while skiing about six months before this last bout of depression began. Her sciatic pain left during this second session.

I'll have a few more appointments with her to make sure that the compression doesn't return. If it does, it means that I didn't find and effectively correct the underlying cause. If the compression doesn't return, it means that the cause most probably was the fall she remembered and that it is now effectively corrected. This lady will probably want to have well-person treatments periodically after this problem is totally resolved. I think it is a good idea. Why wait until we have overt symptoms? Craniosacral system evaluations can frequently uncover a problem before it becomes a symptom. Correction of the asymptomatic craniosacral system dysfunction can avoid the unpleasantness of symptoms.

10

The Famous TMJ Syndrome

Many people are becoming familiar with the TMJ syndrome. ("TMJ" is the abbreviation for temporomandibular joint; "syndrome" is defined as a group of symptoms that characterize a specific disease or problem.) The TMJ syndrome is thus the group of symptoms that are known to relate to functional and sometimes structural problems with the temporomandibular joints. The temporomandibular joints are those joints, located one on each side of your head, that are directly in front of the openings in your ears. They are the joints that allow your lower jaw to go up and down. These joints enable you to open and close your mouth freely and to chew. If you put your index fingers in your ears as though you are trying to block out a loud noise, and open and close your jaw a few times, you can feel this joint moving through the front wall of your ear canal.

The TMJs are very important joints in your body because you use them to bite, chew, talk, breath, and the like. When the TMJs become a problem, a whole syndrome of discomforts may develop. Among these symptoms we find head, neck, upper-back, jaw and tooth pain, as well as visual disturbances, digestive problems, and personality changes such as anxiety, depression and irritability. The TMJs themselves may become quite painful. They may snap, crackle and pop when you open and close your mouth and, in severe cases, your jaw may get stuck in either the open or closed position.

Dentists have been wrestling with this problem for some time. Usually they get reasonable, but not excellent, success. Most dental treatment that I have seen involves the repositioning of the jaws and/or teeth in relation to each other. There is an attempt at the forced remolding of the positions of the structures that are involved in biting and chewing. Some dentists use other techniques to relax the muscles that we use to open and close our mouths. Among these techniques are trigger-point injections, biofeedback, and a host of other approaches that are meant to help you stop clenching your jaws together and stop grinding your teeth at night.

CranioSacral Therapy is becoming recognized by some of the dental community as a valid treatment approach in many, if not all, cases of TMJ syndrome. CranioSacral Therapy is, of course, controversial, but it is producing good results, and results are difficult to argue against even if you disagree with the theory.

Quite naturally, I have a bias and have used CranioSacral Therapy on hundreds of patients who were suffering from and being treated for TMJ syndrome. The treatment approaches that I have seen used by dentists involve a wide variety of dental splints, appliances, tooth reshaping, and so on. By using CranioSacral Therapy we gently help the bones of the skull to remobilize and reposition themselves naturally so that the patient's own self-corrective tendencies are respected. We view the great majority of temporomandibular joint function problems as part of the symptom complex (syndrome) rather than the cause. We don't like to treat symptoms. Part of the fun of CranioSacral Therapy is the search for the underlying cause. Since the temporomandibular joints are seated in the temporal bones of the skull, if these temporal bones are slightly out of position, the temporomandibular joints begin to malfunction. Then the bite goes out of alignment (malocclusion occurs) and it appears that the cause is a bite problem. However, if the temporal bone position and function is corrected first, the bite will frequently correct itself without costly outside intervention. The problem is not solved for the CranioSacral Therapist until the reason for the temporal bone problem is known and corrected.

I had a patient come in about three years ago with severe problems related to the left temporomandibular joint. She had very severe pain in the left side of her face. You couldn't touch the left cheek bone (zygoma) without making her jump with pain. She had headaches and a stiff neck all the time. She had severe left arm and shoulder pain on bad days. About one-third of her days were "bad days." Her son was a dentist. Her son's partner had taken over her case in an attempt to solve the temporomandibular joint problem. This poor lady was getting no relief, and she was wearing one dental appliance at night, a different one in the daytime, and using pain pills like they were going out of style. She wasn't getting any better and was becoming desperate. Her son had heard about CranioSacral Therapy and suggested that she see me before the next phase of the dental treatment plan was instituted. That next phase would have been the reshaping of her teeth in an attempt to reposition her lower jaw.

Craniosacral evaluation revealed the fact that both temporal bones were malpositioned and not moving in accommodation with the rhythmical changes in the fluid pressure within the hydraulic craniosacral system. Further evaluation of the system revealed that the reason for the temporal bones' malfunction was coming from the low back. Here I found that the lower end of the tube of dura mater membrane that connects the low back and pelvis to the skull was suffering a remarkably high and abnormal tension. This problem was stemming from the sacrum, which was malpositioned. This sacrum problem occurred because some of the muscles that attach to it were in an abnormal state of increased contraction. These were the piriformis muscles. She then told me that before all this began she had fainted in her kitchen and fallen to the floor. The reason she had fainted was an overdose of medicine for high blood pressure. I knew now where the TMJ syndrome began. It began with an overdose of blood pressure medication that led to a fainting episode and a fall to the floor. The fall resulted in a twisted pelvis and base of the spine. This twist was maintained because the muscles contracted, as they do, and splinted in order to prevent the injury from getting worse. One of the things I have learned over the years is that many of the mechanisms that protect us and perhaps save our lives in times of emergency begin to damage us later because they don't know when to turn off after the accident is over or the danger is past.

These contracted piriformis muscles were preventing the sacrum at the lower end of her craniosacral system from accommodating the rhythmical hydraulic fluid pressure fluctuations. This condition was also producing an abnormal tension in the dura mater membrane tube up the spinal canal into the head. The membranes in the skull are so arranged that the temporal bones are extremely vulnerable to abnormal tensions in the dura mater membrane system from below. This was the cause of the malposition of the temporal bones. The temporal bone malposition and loss of normal mobility changed the positions of the temporomandibular joint sockets. It made them uneven from one side to the other. The lower jaw bone, otherwise known as the mandible, is a single bone. When the two sockets are not even on both sides of the head, one or the other or both of the temporomandibular joints are stressed. The TMJ syndrome is then set into motion.

I decided to attack this problem from its source. I knew that if I was going to refute all that this nice lady had been led to believe by her dentist son's colleague, I needed a convincing argument. Nothing is more convincing than a dramatic relief of pain. The whole craniosacral system evaluation had taken about 15 minutes. So, without a word, I began work on the piriformis muscles that were binding the sacrum down improperly. This meant that I put one hand under her right buttock, as she lay on her back on the treatment table, and put my other hand on the front and side of the right hip and pelvis. (The piriformis muscles connect the hip and the sacrum.) I could feel her questioning my sanity, although she didn't say a word. I'm sure she was thinking to herself, "Why is this cuckoo working down there? Doesn't he know the problem is up here in my head?" It took about five minutes before the piriformis muscle relaxed. When it did relax, I could feel the sacrum loosen up. I began to encourage and support the sacral movement in accord with the craniosacral system's rhythmical activity. As the sacrum began to move in synchrony with the system, I watched her face relax. At the same time, her body relaxed. She smiled, then began to quietly laugh and cry at the same time. The pain was gone. Her face felt better. Her headache went away. Her neck remained stiff. I went to the left side of her pelvis and released the left piriformis muscle and, with this release, the neck stiffness went away. I didn't have to convince her of anything with words. The results spoke for themselves. She got rid of all her dental appliances and has felt good rather consistently since that first session.

The piriformis muscle needed relaxation training, so I showed her some exercises that would prevent recurrence of the problem. I did follow-up work on the craniosacral system at weekly intervals for about two months. Now I see her about once every three or four months for "tune-up" work and for her peace of mind. She has vivid memories of the pain she endured. This is the craniosacral approach to the TMJ syndrome.

There is another way that the TMJ syndrome can be triggered by dysfunction of the craniosacral system. This is illustrated beautifully by another lady who came to me by recommendation of another patient. She was 58 years of age and had been suffering with severe and episodically disabling headaches and neck pain with numbness in the arms for about 15 years. This patient had been in treatment with her dentist, her chiropractor and her internist for this problem for at least 10 of these years. She had also been in psychotherapy for over six years. She was considering the possibility that the headaches were psychosomatic. She was also being treated for TMJ syndrome by her dentist. She was using "splints" in her mouth to keep her teeth from coming together too tightly and compressing her temporomandibular joints.

Craniosacral evaluation suggested that the top of her head had received a blow or force at some time that forced that part of her skull above the roof of her mouth into a collision with the roof of her mouth. The impact effect had remained. This caused a widening of the roof of the mouth, which in turn produced a malocclusion between the upper and lower teeth. Over the years, this malocclusion and loss of tooth stature resulted in a condition of abnormal wear and tear on the temporomandibular joints. *Voilà*, the TMJ syndrome. In order to solve this problem, I had to lift the skull off the roof of the mouth and then assist the roof of the mouth into a more narrowed position. This treatment process required several hours of work, but it was finally accomplished. This fine lady is no longer using any dental appliance, and she is essentially headache-free—unless she gets very upset about something; then she gets a tension headache as do so many people.

How did this happen? Finally she remembered the cause of the injury. She was a teenager at the time. She was swimming with a group of friends at a lake in Michigan during summer vacation. As she was coming up from underwater next to a raft out in the lake, a young man dove into the water and they met with a lot of head-to-head collision force. She almost drowned. She had to be pulled out of the water and given artificial respiration because she was knocked unconscious. After about 20 years, her ability to adapt to the retained effects of this collision lessened. As her adaptability lessened, the symptoms began. I think she retained a lot of the injury effect because, by being knocked out, some of her self-corrective mechanism was compromised at the time of the accident. We see this happen over and over again.

These solutions are permanent. Both of these patients maintain contact with me, and I know that they are no longer TMJ syndrome sufferers.

11

Chronic Pain and Disability

Another area of healthcare difficulty to which CranioSacral Therapy can and does offer valuable contribution is chronic pain. Chronic pain comes in all shapes and sizes. It is an area that powerfully brings to light the concept of the craniosacral system as the "core" of the person. Chronic pain can be anywhere in the body and for any reason. If it continues long enough, it will affect and compromise the workings of the craniosacral system. If the cause of the bodily pain outside of the craniosacral system is corrected but the craniosacral system is not effectively treated, the pain may continue. This is because the craniosacral system problem remains. These patients frequently end up in psychotherapy or may be considered hopeless. Sometimes the focus of conventional therapy is on teaching them to live with the remaining pain.

Correction of craniosacral system malfunction is often the finishing touch that restores this patient to a normal, pain-free life. This is very often the case in ruptured disc problems. The disc herniation is repaired surgically and the pressure that this ruptured disc was producing on a nerve root is physically removed, but the abnormal tension in the dura mater membrane system remains. This condition of abnormal membrane tension can and does frequently cause the pain pattern to persist from inside the "core" (craniosacral) system, even though the correction has been made outside the craniosacral system. Proper CranioSacral Therapy is often all that is needed to bring the problem to complete resolution.

The ruptured disc is only one cause of pain due to spinal cord nerve-root pressure. This pressure or, more correctly stated, compression may be coming from scar tissue, improperly functioning vertebral joints, abnormal muscle contraction, swollen tissue, calcium deposits, improperly healed bone fractures, and so on. The list is not endless, but it is very long. So many times these problems are correctable; but if the craniosacral system is neglected, the painful symptoms continue. We simply need to remember that painful conditions originating outside of the craniosacral system usually refer into that system. The secondary effect upon the craniosacral system is then frequently powerful enough to continue the pain even though the original cause has been effectively corrected.

Post-Herpetic Neuritis

Recently I evaluated a patient who had suffered from shingles, the onset of which was about four years prior. Shingles, as you may know, is a viral infection of one or more of the nerves that run between the ribs. It is an extremely painful condition. It is accompanied by a skin rash that is excruciatingly painful even when touched by a wisp of cotton. The skin rash follows the course of the nerve. The pattern of the rash is so typical that, coupled with the pain, it is about all you need to make the diagnosis. Shingles rash usually lasts about four to six weeks. Then, if you are lucky, everything subsides and returns to normal. There is usually some residual scar in the skin where the rash was. Before I got into doing CranioSacral Therapy, I had treated a hundred or so cases of shingles using a combination of acupuncture and osteopathic manipulation.

The results were good, but in a small percentage of these patients there was a residual chronic pain left over that responded to nothing that I had found as yet.

This particular patient whom I saw recently continued to have severe pain in the back and around her chest cage between the ribs where the rash had previously been. I had not treated this patient originally. She had been treated with cortisone injections, which got her through the acute phase of the shingles but left her with the chronic pain that had persisted over the past four years. She had received both osteopathic and chiropractic treatment during those years. Both approaches gave incomplete and only temporary relief from pain. The official name for the painful condition she presented to me was "postherpetic neuritis." This condition is estimated to occur and continue for several years after the acute phase in about one out of every 10 cases of shingles (herpes zoster).

As I evaluated this lady's craniosacral system, it became obvious that the dura mater membrane within the spinal canal would not glide freely at the level where the herpes zoster virus had attacked her intercostal nerve. This is the nerve that runs between the ribs and is under the rash. The residual scar of the shingles rash told me precisely which nerve had been involved with the herpes zoster virus attack.

I think what happens is that the inflammation of the involved nerve root moves centralward into the craniosacral system as well as out into the body along the nerve trunk. When we successfully remobilize the craniosacral membrane system inside the spinal canal, the residual pain disappears. This is precisely what happened with this lady. Four years of pain ended within a 40-minute craniosacral treatment session. Why? Because we dealt with the "core" as well as the periphery.

Crushed Pelvis with Severe Craniosacral System Dysfunction

Chet was an inner-city schoolteacher in Detroit when his accident happened. As so many schoolteachers do, he was working construction during the summer break. A cable snapped on a crane and a load of steel rods came plummeting down onto him. Fortunately they landed on his lower body. It is difficult to reconstruct exactly what happened, but Chet ended up lying on his back in the dirt, pinned down by this load of steel rods across his pelvis. His pelvis was fractured in three places.

Subsequent to his accident, and after all the bones had healed, Chet realized that he could not put his thoughts into words easily and quickly as he used to do. As this realization sunk in, he further realized that he wouldn't be able to teach school since he couldn't stand up before a class and express his ideas and thoughts effectively in words. He could talk, but it took time to get the words out. This wouldn't work, especially in the inner city where the students would go for his vulnerability as soon as they saw it. Chet couldn't hide his vulnerability.

In addition to the word expression problems, Chet had lots of low-back and neck pain, headaches, and episodes of unreasonable and difficult-to-control confusion and anxiety.

He was referred to me by an acupuncturist/CranioSacral Therapist about four years after his accident. Chet had reached a plateau in his recovery. They wanted to see if I could move him from his present level of recovery to a higher level of functioning. I really love that kind of a challenge.

Chet was quite intelligent. He had developed skill and success in another profession that did not require much interaction with other people. He was doing quite well in high-risk investments and handicapping sports events. He was very adept with numbers and statistics.

When I saw Chet the first time, he came to Florida for two weeks. I treated him eight times during those two weeks. In my opinion, his meningeal membrane system was bound down tightly in his pelvis due to the injury. Since this membrane system is continuous into the head, the impairment of membrane flexibility and function was passed on into his head and neck from his pelvis. This accounted for the problem with talking, the headaches, neck pain, and episodes of anxiety and confusion.

I began work on his pelvis. In response to this pelvic work, his mental symptoms and head-neck pain began to change. We concluded from this observation of the head changing while I worked on the pelvis that we were on the right track. Chet decided to stick with me.

Today Chet feels good. He has few headaches, his neck is fine, he has no more anxiety, and his speech is about 75 percent improved. Chet has not gone back to teaching, though, because he is doing so well with his investment speculations.

Since I began working with Chet about four years ago, he has returned for a week of treatment about three or four times each year. He continues to improve even between treatment sessions. That's the way CranioSacral Therapy is. It sets the wheels of self-healing in motion. Patients are often better the next time you see them than they were when you finished the last time. Chet is an example of this aspect of CranioSacral Therapy. I think his new plateau will be "normal."

Restoration of Brain Function After Coma
Jean was 62 years of age when she came in for her first appointment. She was one of the most organized people I had ever seen. Everything was written down. Explanations had to be given over and over again. She questioned everything.

Actually she drove my receptionist crazy with her questions before we ever met her.

When she arrived for her first appointment I was astonished. She gave me a long history of coma and disability subsequent to an auto accident about 20 years earlier. She had been told then that she would never walk again. Not only was she walking, but every morning she was swimming 50 laps nonstop in a 30-meter pool. She didn't trust doctors because they had tried to convince her that she would be an invalid for the rest of her life. Had she listened to them, she would have lived "down" to their expectations.

As she appraised me, I could feel her "daring" me to say something negative or pessimistic. Her determination and self-discipline had gotten her back into the mainstream of life, and woe be unto anyone who said the wrong thing to her.

Her purpose in this visit with me was to determine whether or not she wished to have some CranioSacral Therapy. She had noticed that her memory was failing a little. Actually it had failed a lot, and that was the reason for writing everything down. Also, her ability to concentrate and comprehend was less than it used to be. That turned out to be the reason for all the questioning and requesting for repeat explanations. She knew her weaknesses and was not about to be controlled by them.

Jean had heard that CranioSacral Therapy could help brain function. I confirmed that it could, but I also emphasized that I could not make any promises. She said she would let me know. That first appointment was only talk, a real question-and-answer session. Even though it was a bit trying, I felt a deep respect for this woman's tenacity and determination.

In a week or so she called and announced that she would take 10 CranioSacral Therapy treatments at one-week intervals. She felt that 10 sessions should be enough to help her brain function, if indeed this treatment could help.

She did improve greatly. During her 10-week trial period she began to question much less, required only one or two explanations about the same subject in order to comprehend, and stopped writing everything down. Even better, she relaxed a great deal and was much less driven and uptight. She continued to exercise by walking and swimming, but it was not as much a compulsion now as it was a recreational activity.

Now it is seven years later, and Jean comes in for a Cranio-Sacral Therapy session every couple of months. She comes in because it helps her to feel better. She is nice and kind of fun to be with. I enjoy her appointments because each time I see her we have a challenging and lively conversation. Also, I get confirmation of the beneficial power of CranioSacral Therapy.

Spinal Cord Injury

John was a healthy American male when he fell out of a tree. He was at a party that night. He got "high" and decided to show off. He climbed the tree, fell out, and broke his back. That was about three years ago. He was in his mid-30s at the time. He was getting high a lot in those days. He was a promising young playwright. He was living in the fast track.

After John fell out of the tree, he couldn't move his legs nor could he feel them. He soon discovered that he had lost control of his bowel and his bladder. It was devastating. Imagine what it would be like to suddenly be totally dependent, to be losing your bodily waste products without even knowing that it was happening. It would be especially devastating when you are young, single, handsome and showing promise of great success.

John showed up at our two-week intensive program for

brain and spinal cord dysfunction patients. He received very intensive treatment seven to eight hours per day, five days a week for two weeks. This treatment program included everything that is discussed in this book: CranioSacral Therapy, Energy Cyst Release, SomatoEmotional Release, Therapeutic Imagery and Dialogue, as well as individual and group psychotherapy. It also included acupuncture, meditation, physical therapy, occupational therapy, therapeutic exercise, a wide variety of massage therapy approaches and yoga exercises.

By the end of the two weeks, John was beginning to regain control of bowel and bladder function. He was feeling sensations in his legs and lower body, and beginning to be able to move his legs just a little.

It is now two years later. John has worked regularly with one of our CranioSacral Therapists who is a physical therapist. He made significant progress during this time. He returned to our center for treatment one week at a time on three occasions after his first two-week intensive program.

A few months ago, John moved to Florida so that we could have the time to work more intensively. His legs are doing remarkably well. He can move them and walk with assistance now. I fully expect John to walk unassisted.

As I reflect on this case I realize that we are too dumb to know that we are attempting the impossible. So we try and try and try... and sometimes it works.

Expectation plays such a great role in success. Expect defeat and that's what you get. Expect success and that's what you get.

There are upwards of 2,000 cases of chronic, unrelenting pain in our files that have responded favorably to CranioSacral Therapy after many other treatment approaches provided only partial and/or temporary relief.

Disability Prevention

Now let's look at an example wherein I believe we averted the disability of a major stroke. And we taught the husband how to do the work.

Annette was 72 years of age when I met her the first time. She had fallen on the sidewalk just down the street from my offices. Her husband, Harry, had brought her directly into our waiting room. I was able to see her within a few minutes.

Her injuries weren't too bad. She had a right knee that was abraded, bleeding a little, full of tiny stones and dirt particles, and swelling rapidly. She had also fallen on her hip, which was beginning to hurt a lot. I wondered if she might have sustained a fracture. Her right elbow was also cut and swelling rapidly. Her glasses were totally shattered. She had a large bruise on her forehead and on the side of her face. Her blood pressure was 190/110.

In those days I had an x-ray machine in my office, so I took some pictures of her injured areas. There did not appear to be any broken bones. I wanted to be very sure that she hadn't fallen because the hip had fractured spontaneously first. This would cause her to fall. Sometimes this happens. The bones get so brittle that the patient's hip fractures by itself and causes the fall rather than the fall causing the broken hip. In Annette's case there was no fracture anywhere, and her bone density on the x-rays looked pretty good. Harry thought she must have tripped on a seam in the sidewalk. Annette was confused. She had no idea why she had fallen. The more I talked with her, the clearer it became that she most likely "blacked out" for just an instant and fell. This is typical of what we used to call the "small stroke syndrome." Since then it has been named the "transient cerebral ischemic attack." No matter what you call it, the small stroke syndrome or the transient ischemic attack, it's all the same thing. What it means is that, for short periods of time, the brain doesn't get enough blood supply. During these periods of poor or compromised blood flow, the patient experiences confusion, numbness somewhere, loss of control of some parts of the body, or, as in Annette's case, may black out completely for an instant.

As I continued to talk with Annette, she began to admit that she had experienced several episodes of momentary confusion. She described the small stroke syndrome beautifully. The larger concern is that when "small strokes" begin, it is not uncommon that a full stroke occurs shortly afterward. The small stroke is a warning sign.

In addition to some medication to assist the blood flow to her brain, I elected to use some CranioSacral Therapy techniques to further enhance Annette's supply of oxygenated blood into her head. There are three techniques in Cranio-Sacral Therapy that I have found to be extremely helpful to the patient with small strokes: (1) the thoracic inlet release; (2) the occipital cranial base release; and (3) the parietal lift with traction.

I did these techniques three times a week with Annette. Within two weeks her moments of confusion ended. She did not fall again. She liked the CranioSacral Therapy a lot because it made her feel good. She wanted the treatments to continue, but of course Medicare objected to me treating Annette three times a week, so they began to withhold payment. Annette and Harry were living on a pension. They were not wealthy, so I decided to ask Harry if he would like to learn how to do the CranioSacral Therapy techniques for Annette. Harry was eager to learn. He had watched me several times and had seen how gentle and easy CranioSacral Therapy is to do. Harry learned very quickly and took over the hands-on craniosacral treatment of his dear wife. He did the techniques three times weekly, and I saw Annette once a month after that for about three years. Her small strokes did not return.

It wasn't long after Harry began treating Annette that they came in and asked if I could teach Annette to treat Harry. She was feeling so much better, with more energy and alertness, that she wanted to share it with her husband. Annette learned to do some of the treatment for Harry. They were both very happy about helping each other. I'm sure they felt more useful and fulfilled. After about three years Annette and Harry moved back to Wisconsin to be closer to their family, and I lost track of them.

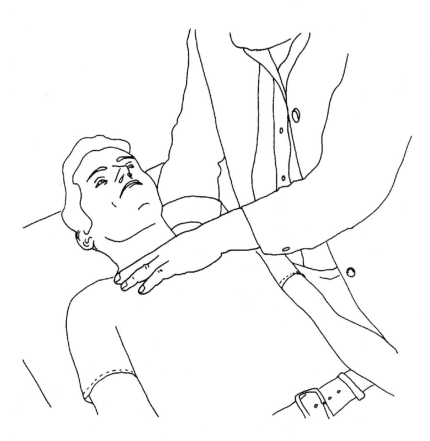

Illustration 5
The thoracic inlet release technique

12

Insights

Our extensive work with chronic pain and other problems has opened the doors to many other insights. Among them are tissue memory, Energy Cysts, SomatoEmotional Release, the power and significance of intention and touch, the use of Therapeutic Imagery and Dialogue and, last but not least, who can do this kind of work. The path just goes on and on. At present I am reasonably convinced that the only limitations imposed upon our self-healing abilities are those that we ourselves construct out of the negative beliefs that we hold about self-healing.

I realize now that my job is as a facilitator to the patient's own healing process. This realization is a long way from my beginnings in medicine when I thought I could "cure" people. I "cured" all kinds of heart attacks, strokes and acute injuries. I really thought it was me who was doing it. I felt guilty, a failure, when one of my patients didn't get well.

Today I know that I was immature and on an "ego trip" during those early days. Today I know that the patient does the healing and that I am privileged to witness and perhaps participate in his or her healing process. Today I know that I am the student and the patient is my teacher. Perhaps you'll understand better what I mean as you read the following chapters.

13

Tissue Memory! What Next?

In working with patient after patient in a one-on-one setting with prolonged, quiet-touch contact as is required when we are doing CranioSacral Therapy, I find my hands almost moving by themselves. My hands move to certain areas of the patient's body wherein there seems to reside some sort of memory of the injury that has occurred. These certain areas may or may not have been related to my intended focus during that particular part of the treatment session. I learned very quickly to give my hands the freedom to go where they seem to be drawn. I still watch in wonderment as my hands lead me to places in the patient's body that I might not have found otherwise.

These places where my hands go are invariably connected somehow to the primary problem. They are connected in a much more basic way than the symptom. Frequently I simply let my hands rest where they have been drawn. As I let them rest, I take on an observer's attitude. Heat usually generates under or between my hands — more heat than either my own skin or the patient's skin is providing. Then there often develops a pulsing activity that I begin to monitor. It is usually a little slower than the patient's heart pulse. We have named this the "therapeutic pulse" because something good seems to be happening inside of the patient while it is going on.

Usually the heat rises to a peak, remains high for a few minutes, and then cools. At the same time that the heat peaks to maximum, the therapeutic pulse crescendos to a stronger amplitude. The rate does not increase. Then the therapeutic pulse decrescendos below my ability to perceive it as the cooling occurs.

Immediately after these phenomena have finished, the patient usually reports a lessening of pain. A perceptible relaxation of body tissues occurs. Frequently, but not always, at this juncture the patient might report feeling some kind of emotion like fear or anger. He or she might also report a rather vivid memory of an accident or injury that is apparently related to this area of the body. The memory doesn't always occur at the time of the tissue release. It may come into the patient's consciousness that night or even a few days later. Sometimes the memory doesn't come, but the patient feels better anyway.

I have come to look upon this phenomenon as "tissue memory." By this I mean that the cells and tissues of the body may actually possess their own memory capabilities. These tissue memories are not necessarily reliant upon the brain for their existence. I feel this way simply because I have been in hundreds of CranioSacral Therapy treatment sessions wherein it seemed that an injury stored in the tissue was released, yet the patient became aware of this incident only after the tissue released heat, went through the "therapeutic pulse" phase (that I described above), and then relaxed and softened.

I presented this concept of tissue memory to a group of physical therapists a while back at one of their annual conventions in New England. There was a rather strong disagreement coming from one member of the audience. She was arguing that it wasn't possible that a tissue, such as a muscle, could actually possess independent memory capability.

She had a rather strong background in psychology and was insisting that somehow I was stirring up the brain memory of the injury. My salvation came from a physicist in the back of the room. This physicist had been researching energy fields for the U.S. Military for 15-plus years. He had come with me to this part of the country to do some joint research. He decided to stay and attend the conference in order to broaden his knowledge. I'm certainly glad he was there, because he saved me an argument about this question of tissue memory that probably would not have reached a satisfactory resolution.

The physicist simply reminded us of the fact that we could store a symphony on something as simple as a piece of plastic tape and a total TV program, complete with color and sound, on something just a little more complex but still of simple plastic. Therefore, he continued, it seemed to make sense that something as complex as a muscle tissue, a bone or a piece of liver could store the memory of an accident or injury. Think about it. The argument ended very abruptly, and I thanked him for his observation.

Just last week (December 1990) I was working with a 40-year-old colleague who had been in an airplane crash in 1974. It was a small plane, and the other two people in the plane died in the crash. He lay in the airplane with a broken back, totally conscious, for two hours before he was found, rescued and hospitalized. His body apparently healed from the effect of the crash, but his lower neck, low back and left leg have been somewhat painful ever since. Over the last year, his left leg has been getting harder to control. It doesn't want to do what he tells it to do, and it has become more painful. He does have a ruptured disc that could be producing the problem, but he wants to avoid surgery if it is at all possible. This man is a doctor and knows that disc surgery has attendant risk. I had treated him once before about six months prior to this present session. He stated that he had improved significantly for about six weeks after that first session. During that initial session I simply used gentle techniques to decompress his back and worked to normalize his craniosacral system function.

On the occasion of this second treatment session, my right hand was drawn very powerfully to his left ankle and foot. I have learned to trust the wisdom of my hands, so I let this hand do whatever it wanted to do. My fingers found some very definite places to locate on the ankle and on the top of the foot. I waited with my right hand on his left foot and ankle. My left hand then found its way to the front of his left pelvis. It felt to me like there was a focus of injury in this area. He denied pelvic fracture, but remembered later that his belly muscle, the abdominus rectus, had been torn away from the pelvis in front and on the left side during the accident. We chatted a while with my hands in place. I waited to see what his body tissues wanted to do. After a few minutes he commented that something was happening in his leg. He didn't know how to describe it. As so often happens in this work, the patient feels something but has no frame of reference. Patients have never felt anything like it before and so initially they may doubt their feelings, probably because the sensations are so new.

In any case, this feeling, which he described as "something" in his leg, corresponded to a softening of the tissues on the front of the pelvis along with a heating up of his left ankle and foot and crescendo of the "therapeutic pulse" in that same ankle and foot. The heat and therapeutic pulse then decrescendoed out of my sensitivity range. I say it this way because I don't know whether the therapeutic pulse totally disappears or whether it just becomes too subtle for my skill levels to perceive. As these changes subsided, he began to move his back and leg in a rather experimental way. It was at this point that he remembered the torn belly muscle. He reported that his back and leg felt "different." I asked if he meant "good" different or "bad" different. It took a few seconds, but he finally said that it felt very good. He got up and walked around a bit. Because he is a doctor, he was cautious in his admission that his condition had improved so dramatically from just an hour's work. Doctors know this is impossible. But if it feels better, why not say it? We don't say it because we are taught that these kinds of changes can't happen. But "seeing is believing."

From my viewpoint, we had released an Energy Cyst from his body. I was working with another physicist when we developed this idea of the Energy Cyst. We were researching the electrical changes that occur in the human body during my kind of treatment approach. This was several years ago, when we were both members of the Biomechanics Department at Michigan State University. The other physicist, Dr. Zvi Karni, marveled at the way I could take the body of an injured person, place it in a very specific position, and get relief from long-standing pain. We began measuring body voltage during treatment. When this body position of pain relief was obtained, the total body voltage of the patient went down very low. As the position of pain relief was maintained, the aforementioned heat release and "therapeutic pulse" would occur. As these (heat and therapeutic pulse) phenomena ended, the patient's total body voltage would go up again, but usually only about half as high as it had been before. This drastic voltage drop occurred only when the treatment procedure was successful. If I was not successful in obtaining lasting pain relief, the patient's voltage would usually return to its previously high level. If I didn't find the exactly correct body position, the voltage wouldn't drop until I did.

Another very helpful thing we discovered at that time was that when the patient was in the exactly correct therapeutic position to release the pain, not only did the patient's total body voltage drop, but the rhythmical activity of the craniosacral system also came to an abrupt and complete stop. If I didn't have the patient in the exactly correct position, the craniosacral system rhythm did not stop. When it did stop, it didn't start again until the heat was released and the therapeutic pulse had decrescendoed out of sight. This is another reason why I think of the craniosacral system as "core" to the total being. It tells me when I'm doing the right thing with the patient.

How do we find the correct position for bodily release of the injury? I honestly don't know. I can describe what I think we do, but we are still wide open to other ideas. As I see it, these body tissues retain memory of the position the body was in when the injury occurred. When I put my hands on the patient's body, I try to silently assure these tissues that we will only do what they want us to do. I also try to think about putting energy into the patient's body. I know this is happening because we have measured voltage rises and resistance reductions in electrical parameters during these treatment sessions. Then I try to be very sensitive and counter the gravitational forces on the patient's body so that tension balances between antagonistic muscle groups can be obtained as though we were in a gravity-free environment. Once this happens, I follow the balance until the craniosacral system abruptly ceases its activity. Then I know that we are in the right place for something good to happen. Initially I was doing all of this intuitively. It has remained for my physicist friends to document scientifically what has been happening.

After we saw the reliable electrical and physiological changes that I have described, the next question that required

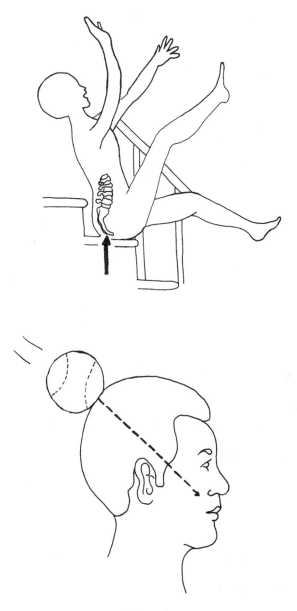

Illustration 6
Arrows indicate direction and penetration of force
as it enters the body during a traumatic experience

attention was: What happens to make the patient feel better? Here my first physicist co-worker and I spent many hours in conversation. I studied physics under his tutelage, and he studied biology, biomechanics and medicine under mine. It was a very rewarding time in my life. It was this physicist, Dr. Zvi Karni, who later brought me to Israel, where we continued some of our unfinished work. Dr. Karni died of a series of heart attacks after his return to Israel. I think of him often.

Back to the question. After much thought-provoking discussion, sometimes friendly and quiet and sometimes quite passionate and heated, we came to agreement on a possible way that this treatment process was having its effect. We designed a model with which we could work. It explained most of the happenings that we were observing and experiencing.

14

The Energy Cyst: A Model

The idea goes like this. When an injury or accident occurs, the energy of this injury or accident enters the body. The laws of thermodynamics tell us that energy cannot be created nor destroyed. They also tell us that the natural tendency of particles (atoms and molecules) and energy is toward disorganization. This disorganization is called "entropy." When external energy is put into your body during an accident or an injury, this energy is in excess of the normal. The usual method of injecting or putting this energy into you is by a blow from something or a collision with something. We decided to call this outside energy the "energy of injury."

When this "energy of injury" is put into you, it penetrates into your tissues to a depth that is determined by the amount of force behind the collision versus the density of the tissues. We can also think of this force as the momentum of the blow. This force or momentum is then dampened or countered by the density or viscosity of the tissues it is trying to penetrate. So a blow on the foot or ankle (such as we saw in our patient who had the airplane crash) might penetrate through the leg all the way to the pelvis. When it reaches its depth of maximum penetration, it stops and forms a localized "ball" of foreign or external energy that doesn't belong there. If your body is vital and able, the energy of injury can be dissipated and normal healing can occur. If your body is unable to dissipate this energy, it (the energy) is compacted into a smaller and smaller ball in order to minimize the area of disruption of tissue function in your body. As the energy of injury is more and more compressed and localized, the disorganization within this compressed energy increases. This becomes an Energy Cyst in your body. This Energy Cyst can and does cause pain and loss of vitality where it resides in your tissues. I have released Energy Cysts from lungs and ended recurrent bronchial infections. On one occasion I released an Energy Cyst from a person's chest and saw normalization of the electrocardiograph and an end to chest pain (angina). These Energy Cysts can come in from a variety of directions and for various reasons. A frequent route of entry for the lungs is through the shoulder. Bladder Energy Cysts frequently result from a fall on the back side. The one I mentioned in the heart came in through a fall from a high place onto the right buttock.

How do we know where the Energy Cyst makes its entry? Because the body, when it is treated in the way I have described, will go to the position it was in when the injury occurred. The heat will exit out of the place where it went in. This heat exit shows you the point of entry.

What makes the body require the precise position for therapeutic release of the Energy Cyst? Dr. Karni and I postulate that the easiest way for the "energy of injury" to exit is the way in which it entered. The path of entry must be straight in order for exit to occur. When the body changes its position after the entry, the path of entry becomes bent. In order for the entry path to become the exit path, it must be straight again. The only way to get the straight path back again is for the body to assume the same position it was in when the injury originally occurred. The tissues remember this position.

They will help you guide the patient's body to the correct position if you, the therapist, are very perceptive and sensitive to the subtleties of the patient's body.

I also think that the energy you supply the patient through your well-intentioned touch (which shows up as voltage increase in the patient) helps to activate that patient's self-correcting mechanisms.

It is possible, after you have gained experience with these techniques, to release Energy Cysts without using the patient's body position as the facilitating factor—but this approach requires a lot more work on your part. It involves using your own energy to overpower the patient's body energy that is walling off the Energy Cyst. This is a much less natural approach. It requires that you judge it worthwhile to over-power the patient's defense mechanism. We must be careful of this overpowering approach. When the therapist overpowers the patient's defenses, it is more likely that mistakes will happen. It is always better to work with the patient's body rather than against it.

15

Back to Tissue Memory and More

During my first teaching expedition in Europe in 1977, I was presenting a seminar to French osteopaths in Paris. It turns out that a very well-known French osteopath, Jean-Pierre Barral, was on the treatment table acting as the subject (patient). The student osteopath was being assisted in learning proper hand placement by my teaching assistant, Monique. It seems that while she was touching his head during the process of hand placement instruction, he got the impression that there was some visceral problem in her body that he would like to further define. He had the interpreter communicate his feeling to me. He further indicated that his examination would not require that he actually touch Monique's body in any way, not even through her clothing.

I described Jean-Pierre's rather strange request to Monique. Both she and I were rather intrigued that this French osteopath would detect a visceral problem in her as she touched him, and that he could further define the problem without actually touching her body or removing her clothing. Monique agreed to the examination. I informed the interpreter, and he assured me that Jean-Pierre was totally honest, ethical and perhaps the most successful osteopathic practitioner in all of France. I was very intrigued. I had graduated from the College of Osteopathy and Surgery in Kirksville,

Missouri; this school was steeped in tradition. I had not encountered anything like that which we were about to be privileged to observe.

Monique was asked to lie on her back on the treatment table fully clothed. Jean-Pierre began moving his hands over her body in circles and short sweeps. His hands remained between six and 18 inches away from her at all times, moving in and out between these distances. Soon he began speaking under his breath softly and to himself. Within a minute or two he began speaking to the interpreter, who gave us a very accurate medical and surgical history of Monique. He spoke about the appendectomy at age 20, the two Caesarean sections in her later 20s, and about her thyroid problem during one of the pregnancies. This was most remarkable in that the whole thing took just a few minutes, and he never touched her. He did miss the fall on her back that fractured her sacrum when she was about 11 years of age. He knew something was wrong there, but he did not know what it was. The problem that initially caught his attention was related to an improper healing subsequent to one of the Caesarean sections. This was later verified as a source of pelvic pain. The verification occurred about five years later during a surgical exploration for this problem.

After he completed his evaluation of Monique, Jean-Pierre invited me to use my own approach to evaluate his body. At that point in the seminar, I was teaching the use of craniosacral system evaluation at the patient's head in order to discover problems in the body. The basis of this technique is the fact that ongoing body problems outside of the craniosacral system ultimately reflect into the craniosacral system and can be discovered there by a skilled evaluator.

I held Jean-Pierre's head and evaluated his dura mater membrane for mobility within the spinal canal. I discovered his stomach problem this way. He became as impressed with my approach as I was with his. We became very good friends. Jean-Pierre and I, along with our families, have spent time together almost every year since this first meeting in Paris. We share our experiences and continually explore together and challenge each other's concepts.

I tell you this story because I believe that, by some means, Jean-Pierre Barral has tuned-in to tissue memory. As I have watched him work over the past years, it has become clear to me that, more often than not, Jean-Pierre does not tune-in to the whole person; rather he tunes-in to a part of that person. It would seem that he becomes oblivious to the whole person and somehow gets information from the tissues or organs upon which he is focused. I know this is a strange concept to consider, but watching Jean-Pierre work, you realize that what he does is also quite out of the ordinary. He communicates with tissues. My intuition says that he is getting his medical and/or surgical history from individual tissues and organs rather than by some psychic or telepathic connection with the patient's mind.

Incidentally, Jean-Pierre teaches what he does quite successfully to serious students. He has come to the United States and given seminars for The Upledger Institute for several consecutive years now. I return the favor and teach seminars in CranioSacral Therapy and SomatoEmotional Release in France quite often also. We both enjoy sharing that knowledge with which we have been presented.

16

SomatoEmotional Release®

SomatoEmotional Release is a term that we have coined to describe a phenomenon that began to occur with great regularity as we became more and more proficient in the use of CranioSacral Therapy and the release of Energy Cysts. SomatoEmotional Release involves the use of body position and energy transference between therapist and client, as does the release of Energy Cysts and tissue memories. The difference lies in the wholism of the approach and the almost complete lack of direction by the therapist.

In the release of Energy Cysts and tissue memories, the therapist has a specific problem in mind that is usually presented as a complaint by the patient. Then, using evaluation techniques such as craniosacral system evaluation and total-body "arcing," the therapist locates the Energy Cysts and makes use of body position and clues from the craniosacral rhythm to release the Energy Cyst. The objective is quite clear during the treatment session.

I should placate your curiosity somewhat at this point and tell you briefly that "arcing" is a method that we have developed that makes use of energy activities in the patient's body. We use these energies to locate the Energy Cysts. Our concept is analogous to what you see when you drop a pebble upon the surface of a rather still pond of water. The waves on top of the water spread out in circles from the point where the pebble entered the water. The waves produced by the pebble's entry interfere with the normal activity of the water in the pond. We find that Energy Cysts in the patient's body send out similar waves of interference in an otherwise normal sea of energy. CranioSacral Therapists can and do develop the perceptual skill to discover these waves of interference produced by the Energy Cysts. We then follow these circular waves to their center, and there it is—the Energy Cyst.

In SomatoEmotional Release, the approach is quite different. Here we simply place our hands on the patient. We then give silent permission for the patient's body to do whatever it deems appropriate at the time. We offer to put energy into the patient. Before you get excited about my "craziness" for speaking so matter-of-factly about "putting energy into the patient's body," understand that we have measured very prominent changes in body voltages, as well as changes in electrical resistance, in both therapist and patient when this "energy" is offered by the therapist and accepted by the patient. We are collecting more and more documented measurements that relate to this "energy transference" phenomenon. When we have enough, we will present it to the scientific community. True craziness would be to present our concepts and the supporting data too soon, before the experimental foundation is rock solid.

Back to SomatoEmotional Release. We find that when the therapist offers a comforting and trustworthy attitude, the patient is encouraged on some nonconscious level. When we combine conducive attitude with the measurable physical energy of which I spoke earlier, it usually takes only a few minutes for the patient to assume the body position of their choice. I, as therapist, have made no suggestion of specific objective. The choice of what to do during this treatment ses-

78

sion is made by the patient. I try to let him or her know that I support the wisdom of his/her choice and will facilitate or assist in any way that I can.

Once the SomatoEmotional Release begins, the cranio-sacral system activity shuts down, just as it did during the Energy Cyst Release. The SomatoEmotional Release process is, however, more global. The body position allows a generalized release of stored-up emotion. This release seems to come from the body tissues. It is most often expressed through the nervous system, the vocal apparatus, etc. There may be crying, shaking, sweating, laughing, pain...almost anything you can imagine. It all depends on what it is that the patient has non-consciously decided to deal with during that session. I suspect very strongly that there is an inner wisdom within the patient that takes into consideration his or her impression of the therapist's skill. With this in mind, the session is tailored to suit the patient's needs as well as the therapist's ability and dedication. I have felt tested in terms of skill, sincerity and motivation by patients during almost every SomatoEmotional Release treatment session in which I have been involved— and there have been thousands of such sessions so far in my professional career.

SomatoEmotional Release, when it is effective, changes people's lives tremendously. It is as though it gives them a chance to see objectively what they are doing with their lives and how they can change for the better. It gives them recall of experiences, traumas, accidents and the like that they have been holding beneath the surface of their awareness for years. Once these suppressed experiences break through the surface, the problems can be dealt with and resolved. When the problem remains suppressed, it can cause trouble, but you don't know what the cause of the trouble may be, nor do you know the reasons for the symptoms.

As an example of the power of the SomatoEmotional Release process, I shall describe for you a situation that occurred more than 10 years ago. It was a most unlikely occurrence in that the patient was a psychiatrist. He volunteered to come forward from an audience of over 200 healthcare practitioners. I was to demonstrate the technique used to induce the SomatoEmotional Release process, and I needed a patient. I began with him standing next to a treatment table on a stage in a rather large auditorium. I simply placed my hands on his hips as I kneeled on one knee in front of him. This is one of several approaches that we use to begin the process. Almost immediately he began to teeter toward his right side. I eased him onto the floor using my body to support him. He began screaming and cursing in a very loud voice. In order to keep his process going, I simply maintained contact with his left hand and wrist. He continued this "R-rated" performance for about 25 minutes. His body jerked and flopped about like a fish out of water. He did not attempt to take his left hand/wrist away from my grasp. As the process continued, his voice got higher and his screaming and cursing became more and more childlike. Finally he began to cry as a child while he assumed a quiet resting position on the floor. His knees were pulled up toward his chest. I continued to hold his left hand and wrist. After he had cried in this infant way for about five minutes, his body suddenly relaxed. He came back to the here and now. He looked around at all of his friends and associates who had witnessed this demonstration. He appeared somewhat embarrassed.

I asked him if he would like to lie down on the treatment table and allow me to do a few CranioSacral Therapy relaxation techniques in order to end the session in a more balanced mode. He did. As I worked with his head, I asked him if he knew what had happened. He did. He shared with us (all 200-plus of us) the fact that he had been in psychotherapy as a patient for over 10 years. He had also been a practicing psychiatrist for over 13 years. He had been at a "stuck" place in his psychotherapeutic process for about three years. In this stuck place he constantly felt very angry at his father. He had, until that day, been unable to get to the cause of this anger. During this demonstration session, he had re-experienced a time when he was about 1 year old and living in Washington, D.C., where his father was involved in the federal government. He was in a baby carriage. His father was taking him for a walk on a pleasant Sunday morning. He could feel the sun shining warmly down upon him as he lay happily and contentedly in his carriage. All the world was right. His father was with him and he was the center of his father's attention.

Then his father stopped to speak with an acquaintance whom they happened to encounter during their walk. The conversation between his father and the acquaintance went on and on and on. The 1-year-old, someday to be a psychiatrist, was no longer the center of his father's attention. He began to feel neglected. After all, this was his time with his father. Someone was taking it away from him. That someone could divert his father's attention from him so easily was a very hurtful realization. He started to make baby noises. Daddy didn't pay attention; he was deep in conversation by now. Baby became frustrated because Daddy just kept on talking and didn't pay attention to his baby noises and movements. Frustration led to anger. Baby began to cry in full-blown anger. His father reached down into the carriage, grasped baby's left wrist, and said, "If you don't shut up, I'll break your damn arm." Not a very diplomatic statement, but things like this happen.

In the here and now, the demonstration volunteer could

understand how his father may have become involved in a very important and perhaps intense conversation. He could understand also that his father wanted to complete this conversation. Baby kept vying more and more strongly for attention. Finally father ran out of patience, grasped his son by the left wrist and uttered the threat about breaking his arm if he wasn't quiet. Put in context, the knowledge that his father had uttered the threat about breaking his arm if he wasn't quiet didn't seem quite so bad. This patient had knowledge that his father had never physically or intentionally emotionally abused him, so the psychiatrist was better able to accept the idea that his father simply ran out of patience with him at that particular time. True, his father's actions and words were unduly harsh for a 1-year-old child, but his father wasn't perfect, nor was he excessively violent. He was a mortal human being. The psychiatrist could accept that now that he knew what it was about.

The memory of this incident had been suppressed by the patient's consciousness. It was retained in his left wrist. When meaningful contact was made with his wrist by my hand, the recall of the experience was liberated. The patient could then resolve the issue that had been producing an ongoing sense of anger toward his father since the time of the incident. In my opinion, the years of psychotherapy identified the emotion of anger as chronically present. Psychotherapy also illuminated the focus of the anger as being the father. However, after several years of work, the cause of the anger had not yet been identified. It remained for a 40- to 50-minute SomatoEmotional Release demonstration session before an audience of over 200 colleagues to define and resolve the remainder of this problem.

I received a thank you letter from this man about three months later in which he stated that his feelings toward his father had changed significantly for the better.

Another illustration of the power of the SomatoEmotional Release process came in 1979 in Paris. I was lecturing to an auditorium full of skeptical and rather unfriendly French physiotherapists. There were well over 300 of them in attendance. It was requested that I demonstrate how the SomatoEmotional Release process works in practice after I had talked about it at some length. I finally agreed to do so, somewhat against my own better judgement.

Immediately, a middle-aged, rather muscular and obviously macho Frenchman came marching down to the front of the auditorium. It was obvious that I was to demonstrate on him. My interpreter, who was also my friend, warned me that this man was the very vociferous leader of the highly skeptical faction in the audience who was saying that this was all "hogwash." I found myself in a rather difficult position. I was discussing concepts that are rather intangible. I had an audience that was grumbling about what I was trying to present. And now I had to demonstrate the practical application of the SomatoEmotional Release process on a big, strong, macho guy who was bragging that he would show me that nothing would happen with him.

I didn't have a treatment table and didn't intend on demonstrating anything. This was to be a morning of didactic lecture. He came to the front of the room. We said "bon jour," which was about 50 percent of my total French-speaking ability. He glared at me in defiance, daring me with his eyes to be so presumptuous as to even dream that this Somato-Emotional Release process could affect him in any way. I placed my hands on the front of his pelvic bones. (For the anatomists, I held his iliac crests and the anterior superior iliac spines.) I went down on one knee as though I was eyeballing the levelness of his pelvis. I said a little prayer begging for success. I silently affirmed my faith in the SomatoEmotional Release process. I put energy into him. It was that generic sort of energy that is offered for whatever use the patient deems advisable at the time.

It is a little difficult to estimate time with true accuracy because in this situation a minute seems like an hour. But I would guess that within 30 seconds this defiant Frenchman fell forward over my right shoulder as though I was to carry him away somewhere. I followed my intuitive sense of what his body wanted to do. I gently lowered his body to the floor in the front of the auditorium. As he slid to the floor, he assumed the fetal position. His knees were on his chest and his thumb was in his mouth. He was crying or sobbing rather mournfully as though he was a very sad and heartbroken little baby. I let him do that as long as he wanted. He seemed aware of the audience and of his colleagues watching him, but as happens in SomatoEmotional Release, he didn't care. His macho braggadocio pride must have diminished in importance at this time.

After about 15 minutes of rather pitiful sobbing and crying on the floor, he stopped rather abruptly. His body relaxed. He acknowledged my presence and began speaking in French to the interpreter. The gist of what he said was that he realized he felt deserted by his mother when he was a baby. He had an older brother who was injured in a bicycle accident. She suddenly had her attention diverted from him to his brother, who had become a disabled child. He could forgive now that he understood. He could stop feeling sorry for himself. I never saw this man again, but I suspect that he was much less macho after this SomatoEmotional Release experience. His excessive macho persona was probably overcompensation for feeling deserted and unloved as a baby. It would be difficult for a baby to understand if suddenly the apparent love and attention that he was used to receiving was significantly reduced. The baby would then need to protect himself from further hurt. Many of us protect ourselves by being tough.

This demonstration further affirmed my faith in the SomatoEmotional Release process. I knew that somebody up there was watching out for me. Since this particular presentation, my acceptance and reception as a teacher and lecturer in France has been most warm and friendly. This macho Frenchman was very influential in the French physiotherapist community.

What made these two rather prominent healthcare professionals go into a deep therapeutic process at the risk of personal embarrassment and in front of hundreds of their colleagues? I don't know. I can tell you that it has happened over and over again. I do three or four demonstrations during each SomatoEmotional Release seminar that I teach. There are about 40 or 50 students in each seminar, and I've been teaching about 10 of these seminars per year for at least five years, and about five per year for the previous five years. So I could guesstimate that I have taught at least 75 seminars with at least three demonstrations during each seminar. This comes to a very conservative estimate of 225 demonstrations in front of classes of 40 or 50 students. Then there have been at least another 50 demonstrations in lecture settings with much larger audiences, many of these in foreign countries. Perhaps I'm suppressing, but I can't think of a single demonstration where nothing happened. I can only think of a few that left much to be desired. Remember, when we begin neither I nor the demonstration patient have any idea what might happen. I do indeed trust the SomatoEmotional Release process, and with good reason.

I think that what happens is that we all live with a sort of "censor" in us that rather paternalistically keeps certain memories and experiences out of our conscious awareness. The intentions of this censor are good. It feels that it is protecting us. However there is an ongoing cost to keeping these memories and experiences beneath the surface. This cost can be manifested as pain, disability, unhappiness, chronic anger, irritability, lack of self-esteem, and so on.

The "censor" considers it worth the cost to keep the memories and experiences buried. There is another part of us which I shall tentatively name the "efficiency expert." The efficiency expert dreams of what life would be like if all of these censored memories and experiences could be brought to the surface, dealt with and resolved. SomatoEmotional Release enlists the body to help the efficiency expert. When we therapists align ourselves with the efficiency expert (who wants to rid the patient of the problems that are hidden beneath the conscious awareness and/or stored in tissues and Energy Cysts as memories and emotions), the censor relaxes, and a positive treatment effect is obtained. I suppose we might say that our energy and presence assists that part of the patient that wants to totally heal the problems rather than just cope with them day by day.

I have described for you a couple of rather sensational types of SomatoEmotional Release experiences. I would like to describe for you now how this process works on a day-to-day basis, one-on-one with patients as they come into the clinic.

I am reminded of a young lady who was referred by a rather prominent psychiatrist because he could find no help for her. She was a highly ranked tennis professional who had developed tennis elbow. She had to drop out of tournament play because the elbow continued to disrupt her ability to play. The referring doctor had used every treatment mode he could think of without satisfactory results. He could obtain some relief, but not enough to allow her to return to the sport that she "loved." (Well, maybe she loved it. We shall see.)

During our first appointment (she was to be with us for a week and see me four times during that week), I realized that there was a connection between the right elbow and her pelvis. I mentioned this possibility to her. She became rather defensive and denied any problems with her pelvis. I didn't disagree with her out loud because the development of a patient-therapist adversarial situation is usually not therapeutically productive unless used as a tool to help the patient express anger or something similar. I did not want to be her adversary as yet, so I allowed her to interpret my silence as agreement that the pelvis probably was not related to the tennis elbow.

On the second day I asked her to stand with her back to me so that I could check her leg length. She agreed to that after I told her I had to work with the foundation as well as with the elbow. This assurance on my part allowed her defenses ("censor") to relax. I'm sure that her "efficiency expert" also knew that there might be an opportunity for a suppressed problem to surface, express and perhaps resolve. I always try to let the efficiency expert know that I'm a friend by the way I touch the patient and by my nonverbal demeanor and intent.

As I placed my hands over the back part of her pelvis and low back, I could feel her beginning to tilt forward. I was not pushing, only touching. I could feel her natural defenses fighting against falling on her face. So I asked her to bend forward, which she did. Her body seemed to like the forward bending. I then asked her to place her hands on the floor so that she was essentially "four-legged" on her feet and hands. Her body liked that idea too. As I asked her to go down on her hands and knees, her craniosacral system stopped pulsing. It remained at a standstill while she was on her hands and knees. I had a strong intuitive sense to place my right hand over the bone in the right side of her pelvis. (This is the bone you sit on, called the ischium.) As soon as I touched this bone, she began to cry and sob. She then went face down on the floor. I maintained my contact with her right ischium. She cried and cried for a long while, fully 15 or 20 minutes. Finally her body relaxed, and her craniosacral system recommenced its rhythmical activity. She smiled through very wet eyes as she looked over her shoulder at me and asked if she could get up.

I asked her to lie down on the treatment table and began to do some gentle, relaxing CranioSacral Therapy techniques aimed at gaining her trust and friendship. I then suggested that if she wanted to talk about anything, I was there to listen.

The story goes like this. About three years before the tennis elbow took her out of play, she had been competing in a national tournament. She had won her game that day but had not played well enough to please her coach. There was an argument between her and her coach out on the tennis court late at night when no one else was around. He was yelling and berating her very severely. She remembered (or seemed to remember) and actually heard his exact words. She turned away from him and began to walk toward the exit gate. He came up behind her and pushed her on the back so hard that she went down on her hands and knees. Then he kicked her in the right buttock so hard that a crack fracture of the right ischium resulted.

This fracture was interpreted as a stress fracture by the doctor. She took about a year off from her intense training and competition. As her coach began to pressure her to get back into a full training program and to compete in the major tournaments, she began to develop the tennis elbow, which simply got progressively worse. Until that day, she honestly believed that the tennis elbow was a valid and separate problem. Now she knew that the tennis elbow was there to prevent her from returning to full-scale competition. She did not want to find herself in the same kind of situation again—a situation that resulted in her coach becoming so angry that he would yell at her, berate her, push her down and kick her. She couldn't stand any more of that. The coach was her father, and he was trying to live vicariously through her because he was never a champion. His joy and his frustration had been through her. From now on, she would live her own life.

In less than an hour, using the SomatoEmotional Release process, she came to all of this realization and insight. She did give up tennis. She discovered that she really didn't like it that much anyway. It was her father who was obsessed with being a champion, not her. During the next two sessions we released a lot of related tissue memories and Energy Cysts. We talked a lot about living for herself and declaring independence from her father. We also talked a lot about his problems, and she developed a sense of empathy and compassion for him. Kind feelings toward her father began to replace the anger and resentment that surfaced during our work. All in all, it was an excellent therapeutic and self-realizing experience for her and for me. Her "efficiency expert" must have been extremely happy, because this whole thing happened in four sessions of about 45 minutes each.

Another wonderful success for SomatoEmotional Release came in the form of a young woman who had been involved in a rather severe automobile accident. She was not really disabled, but she had suffered constant pain during the eight months ensuing the accident. She had fractured three ribs, sustained a whiplash in the neck, and fractured her pelvis. All of her fractures were healed, but she was left with severe headaches that occurred almost daily and were only relieved by several drinks in the evening. The headaches came on during the day as she went about her housekeeping and yard chores. Her neck hurt all the time, as did her back down at the lower end of the rib cage. Her older brother was driving the car when the accident occurred. Though she was unmarried and had never been pregnant, she made no secret of the fact that she liked having a lover at all times. She almost seemed to brag about it.

I saw this young lady a few times and tried very hard to come up with some structural reason in her bones, muscles and ligaments that would account for the severity of the constant pain and the daily intermittent headaches. I found a few things that we corrected, and there was some relief but not much. I cleared the restrictions in her craniosacral system. This helped a great deal with the neck pain, and the headache improved concurrently, but the pain in the middle of her back continued unrelenting. I put her in the sitting position on several occasions and tried without success to induce a SomatoEmotional Release process. She just sat there stiffly and talked about how bad the pain was. I kept telling myself week after week (I saw her once a week) to trust the process. I have since learned that in a case like this it is more effective to see the patient several days in a row. It seems that the increased frequency of treatment sessions inhibits the reorganization of defenses.

In any case, during the 10th session I had her sitting on the treatment table with her back to me. I had one hand on the painful area of her back and the other on the top of her head. I was carefully testing her spine for very subtle movements and, at the same time, pleading for a breakthrough into the SomatoEmotional Release process. My wish was granted. Suddenly she began to push very hard with her back against my hand. The way we respond to this kind of pressure from a patient is to give them an equal amount of resistance to work against. I did this. The harder she pushed, the harder I resisted so that she could not bend backward.

Gradually I saw my hand turn into a fist. Now she was pushing against my fist. Then she screamed and cursed at someone whom I was representing. She told that person to keep his nose out of her business and called him an S.O.B. I went along with this process for a while, saying nothing except to encourage her to keep going. After a few minutes she slumped forward and exclaimed, "Holy s —." I asked her what was going on.

She explained that when she was 13 years old she missed curfew one night, and her mother (who was an alcoholic) locked the doors so that she (the patient) was out all night. She rode her bicycle around for a while and met a man in his 20s who talked to her. He invited her to his apartment and she had her first sexual experience. She did this out of defiance to her mother. A few days later when she and her brother were alone, she told him what had happened. He became very protective and angry. They argued. He hit her with his fist right in the middle of the back where she had been pushing against my fist. The presence of my fist, and the resistance that I offered her, enabled her to simultaneously release the energy of the blow from her brother and the energy of the injury from the car accident that fractured her ribs.

I believe that had her brother not hit her in the back first, she would have probably healed the ribs and the injury of the accident without residual pain. However, something else needed to be released from these tissues. As the release occurred, the memory of her brother hitting her, and her response to it, came flooding back. Next came the realization that, since that time, in order to show her brother he was not her boss, she had sex with a continuous string of men. These men were always older than she by at least 10 years. The coincidence that her brother was driving the car when they had the accident gave her nonconscious mind the opportunity to link her previous (and denied) feelings about her brother to the accident. She then nonconsciously used this opportunity to continue her pain until something was done that allowed her to see how she was using her own sexuality to defy her brother rather than to satisfy her own sex drives and needs for a loving relationship.

Subsequent to this treatment session when the Somato-Emotional Release came through, her whole life turned around. In about a month, her pains were minimal. There was some more releasing to do within the craniosacral system in order to clear the residue of the accident on a physical as well as emotional level, but all things considered she did very well.

It should be pretty obvious by now that CranioSacral Therapy leads to and is intimately related to therapeutic work with tissue memory, Energy Cyst discovery and release, and SomatoEmotional Release. The next integration of this therapeutic approach that occurred was with Therapeutic Imagery and Dialogue. I think it will be very easy for you to see what a valuable adjunct this work has become and how well it fits into CranioSacral Therapy, SomatoEmotional Release and the rest. But first I want to say a few words about the use of the "direction of energy" and then about the power of touch and intention.

17

The Use of Healing Energy

This is a very difficult topic to discuss without loss of credibility. It is so simple that it is hard to believe. I first heard about "direction of energy" as a technique called "V-spread" that was described by William G. Sutherland, an osteopath from the first half of the 20th century who had decided that cranial bones could move. He was not able to prove it to the satisfaction of modern science, but he did become the founder of cranial osteopathy. Sutherland developed techniques to diagnose and treat the joints (sutures) between skull bones that were "stuck" for one reason or another. His focus was mostly on bone, while ours in CranioSacral Therapy is on the use of bones as handles to get beyond into the dura mater membrane system and the hydraulics of the craniosacral system. Dr. Sutherland used his two hands to direct energy from one side of the skull to the other through a stuck suture. He felt that the energy he was directing was recruited somehow from the patient's cerebrospinal fluid and directed into the suture by his hand positions. The suture that was stuck was then mobilized by this energy, and skull-bone motion was restored.

We have found that you do not need the presence of cerebrospinal fluid between your hands in order to direct or focus a "healing energy." We have also seen that this "direction of energy" can be effectively used anywhere in or on the body. We have taught mothers to use it on their children. We have taught parents and loved ones to use it on each other, and we have taught strangers to use it on each other.

What is it? I don't know. I do know that, when it works, it moves the instruments that we use to measure electricity. I know that, when it works, the previously mentioned heat release occurs and the previously described "therapeutic pulse" crescendos and decrescendos. I know that during the time that it is working, the craniosacral system comes to a standstill. What is it? It don't know, but it works.

One of the best examples I can give you is a personal one that I experienced several years ago while I was on faculty at Michigan State University. It was a Saturday morning in late summer. I was out pruning some of the bushes in our rather wild yard. As I cut one branch, another snapped back very fast and hit me in the left eye much more quickly than my reflex could close my eye. I couldn't see a thing with that eye as soon as the branch hit it. Within seconds the pain was absolutely excruciating. I tried hard to see out of the eye, but all I got was light and blurred images. I immediately thought of blindness in my left eye, perhaps losing the eye, needing a corneal transplant, and so on. I controlled my tendency to panic. I made my way back to the house and asked my wife, Dianne, to look into my eye and tell me what she saw. She described an indentation right across the pupil that probably came from the branch striking me. I didn't want to go to the emergency room just because I have worked in emergency rooms myself. I didn't want to plug myself into the conventional healthcare system at this point. This hesitation was probably a manifestation of my own fear about what I might be told.

I went into the bedroom and lay down on the bed to think about this situation. I asked Dianne to please leave me alone for a while. She knew that I meant it and that I was OK. She did leave me alone. I can imagine what the poor woman was going through out in the living room while she waited. After a minute or so of lying quietly on the bed, feeling the pain, and realizing that the vision in my left eye was certainly not improving, I said to myself, "OK, Upledger, you dumb jerk, you teach this direction of energy stuff all the time. Don't you believe what you teach? Don't you practice what you preach?" I embarrassed myself by my poor demonstration of belief in my own doctrine.

I looked at the clock with my good eye. The time was 11:22 a.m. I put my right hand on the back of my head. The fingers of this hand would be the "sending fingers." I used the index, middle and ring fingers for this purpose. I cupped my left hand over my left eye so that I would be looking into the palm of my hand (if I could have seen with that eye). Then I started concentrating on sending energy from my right hand at the back of my head to my left hand in front of my left eye. It took a few minutes to get it started. It probably took a little extra time because I had to detach from myself in order to focus my attention on the sending of energy rather than on the fantasies of what life would be like without a left eye. Would I wear a patch? Would I get a false eyeball? All of these things were running through my head. And man, did this thing hurt.

After I got my concentration and focus working for me, the eyeball began to pulsate. I sensed that this was the "therapeutic pulse." As the pulse crescendoed, I became aware of heat radiating out into the palm of my left hand. I allowed my fingers to reposition themselves on the back of my head any way they wanted to. As the pulse amplitude built and the heat increased, the pain in the eye got worse and worse. A few times I considered stopping because it hurt so much. But I

95

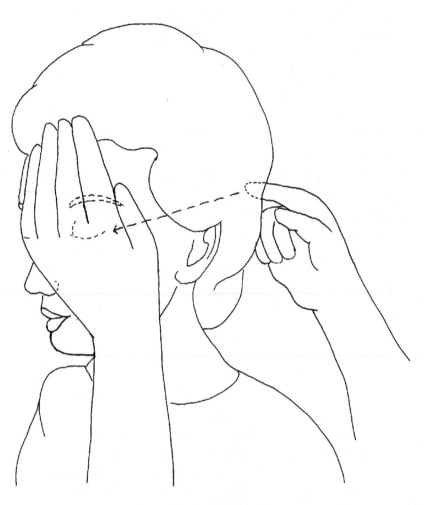

Illustration 7
V–spreading the eye

didn't stop because I wanted to "practice what I preach"; plus the detached part of me was very interested to see what the outcome would be. I vacillated back and forth a few times, but in the end I was very happy that I kept on going with the direction of energy.

Suddenly there was "pop" in my eyeball. I was sure that pop could have been heard out in the living room. In retrospect I'm not sure there was any sound at all except inside my skull. But at the time, I guarantee that I heard it loud and clear in my own head. Right after the pop, the pain went away. All of my panic and fear disappeared, and I could clearly see the palm of my hand with my left eye. I exclaimed to myself, "Wow, this stuff really works!" The time was 11:30 a.m. This whole treatment took a total of eight minutes.

I went out into the living room smiling. Actually I was trying hard to be "cool." What I wanted to do was jump for joy. I had no pain, I could see, and this stuff I teach works on me, too. I asked Dianne to look at my eye again. She couldn't find the dent across the pupil. I had no after-effect from the eye injury. To myself, so as not to appear too crazy, I thanked the bush for providing this opportunity for me to confirm the efficacy of the direction of energy technique. I'm sure that I released an energy cyst from my eye that had been put there by the branch. I also believe that some healing energy was provided from somewhere.

A few more examples of how direction of energy can be used may be helpful. I'm going to give you examples of this technique being used by persons other than myself so that you don't get the idea that I am a singularly gifted person. Direction of energy usage is teachable, and the trainee does not need any background in a healthcare profession in order to use it. The Upledger Institute sponsors a one-day workshop called ShareCare[sm] for laypersons. The attendees are people from all walks of life who want to help others as well as themselves. Direction of energy is one of the things we offer in this one-day workshop.

I once received a phone call from one of the ShareCare attendees named Arthur. He told me that he was up in North Carolina meeting with the governor regarding some tax maneuvers that would save the state money on the buildings it used for state utilities. Arthur was a very successful tax lawyer from Miami. The governor had a bursitis of the shoulder that was causing a lot of pain during the meetings. Arthur offered to put some energy through it to see if it would help. The governor agreed. Arthur did his thing as he had learned how to do it in the one-day ShareCare program. The governor's shoulder pain went away. Arthur felt empowered. The governor felt better but also confused because Arthur is a lawyer, not a healthcare practitioner. We feel good because we believe that we are all born with the natural gift to help each other heal. Arthur's experience offered confirmation. We would like you to use this innate ability. We helped Arthur and the governor to discover that they could heal each other. Organized medicine has taken that gift away from the lay public to some extent through self-aggrandizement and intimidation.

Another example of the use of healing energy by one of our students is much more dramatic and compelling. This student was a nurse's aide in a Chicago hospital. He came on duty on the afternoon shift one day, and there was an elderly lady in one of his assigned rooms who had had her lower leg amputated that morning. She was diabetic and had developed gangrene. It was either lose the foot and lower leg or die. When our student came on duty at 4:00 p.m., this patient was moaning with pain. She was not allowed to have any more morphine until 6:00 p.m. because it was ordered every four hours. She had received her last injection of morphine at 2:00 p.m. The amputation had been completed shortly before noon. There was a light plaster cast on the stump of the leg and up over the knee. Our student was having a hard time listening to this poor lady moaning with pain. He decided he would try this crazy direction of energy technique that we had presented in the introductory CranioSacral Therapy class.

He reports that he held the stump between his two hands and thought about passing a healing energy between them. He imagined the energy going right through the plaster and the stump of her leg between his hands. He felt the "therapeutic pulse" and the heat release. The moaning increased for a minute or so, then it stopped. The patient relaxed and went to sleep. She slept through the rest of his shift until midnight. The next afternoon when he came to work, the records reflected that she had slept through the night. A morphine shot had been given at 9:00 a.m. The records indicated that she had had a good day and was bright and cheerful. She was fine when he saw her a little after 4:00 p.m. that day. She didn't require anymore shots of morphine during her entire hospital stay. He did the direction of energy treatment daily at about 4:30 p.m. and around 11:00 p.m. She was discharged healed and happy about 10 days after surgery. This was quite a remarkable recovery for an elderly, diabetic lady who had her leg amputated because of gangrene. He never told anyone at the hospital, even the lady, what he was doing because they probably would have fired him as a crazy person even though his patient did extremely well.

All of us who have studied CranioSacral Therapy, along with many laypersons who have taken our one-day ShareCare workshops, are helping others, each other and ourselves using direction of energy techniques. Don't knock it until you've tried it. The worst thing that can happen is nothing. The best thing that can happen is that you facilitate healing. Why not try it before you decide that it can't work?

Some years ago I was teaching this direction of energy technique at the Menninger Foundation in Topeka, Kansas. They suggested that it was a form of hypnosis, so they had me do it on babies and animals. It worked. That ruled out hypnotic suggestion. Now let's look at the power of intention along with touch.

18

Intention and Touch

One of my very first beliefs in intention developed in the late '60s when I was beginning to use a lot of acupuncture. At that time we had a free clinic in Clearwater and another in St. Petersburg. Acupuncture was a particularly attractive treatment approach for us because it was cheap and did not involve the use of drugs. Many of our patients were or had been active drug abusers, so the fewer pills we used the better. I saw that some of us could do acupuncture with great success and others didn't get the same degree of success, even on the same patients. At first I thought it was suggestion, so we tried to control any positive or negative comments about expectation. We even went so far as to say nothing at all to the patient before, during or after the treatment.

The strong correlation seemed to be in the unspoken attitude of the therapist. Those of us who had seen acupuncture work and believed in it got much better results than those who did not necessarily believe or disbelieve that it would work. There were two doctors who did it but thought that it was absolute "poppycock." They didn't get good results at all. I often treated the same patient the very next day and got positive results immediately. It was easy to test acupuncture in this way because results for the things we were treating occurred before our eyes during the treatment session. Pain went away.

Breathing in asthma and emphysema patients improved immediately. Cravings for certain addictive drugs like heroine subsided before our eyes. The red-hot rash of shingles faded as we watched when the treatment was done correctly and by a doctor who had confidence in acupuncture. The saying became, "It isn't where or how you put the needles in, it's who puts them there that counts."

This was the beginning of my realization that the attitude and intention of the therapist have a great deal to do with the outcome of the treatment—and this seems to be more than just the power of suggestion. Surgeons who are in a good mood or usually happy seem to get better results than chronically angry, cynical or depressed surgeons. This goes beyond the surgical technique.

Hands-on therapists who are happy, trusting and confident get better results than those who are not. We have begun to measure the effect of attitude upon electrical resistance in a circuit created between the therapist and the patient. We see that higher electrical resistance correlates to negative attitude in the therapist as well as the patient.

Sister Anne Brooks

It was about 20 years ago when I first met Sister Anne Brooks. She had cancelled three appointments and finally showed up for the fourth one.

Sister Anne had applied for work as a volunteer at our St. Petersburg (Florida) Free Clinic. It seems that she wanted to work again with very needy people, and she had heard that our clinic serviced the kind of people whom she wanted to help.

A young man named Butch, who was involved in our Free Clinic program as the director, had interviewed her and suggested that she see me. It seems that she had been struggling with what was diagnosed as rheumatoid arthritis for almost 20 years prior to the interview. At the time of the interview with Butch, it had been recommended by her doctors (there were several in agreement) that she have both of her hip joints surgically replaced with artificial ones. She had been dependent upon a wheelchair for some years before our meeting. The hips had interfered with her walking for about 17 years.

Butch told her that if she wanted to work in our Free Clinic, she would have to see me about her hips. He told her that I did some rather offbeat things like acupuncture, hypnosis, osteopathic manipulation, some strange stuff where you moved skull bones around, and a fairly good brand of general medicine. Fear was a contributing factor in the cancellation of her first three appointments.

When we finally met and I listened to her story, I was touched. She had been the principal at a ghetto school for some years and loved it very much. As her disability and pain worsened, she was transferred to a school that serviced mostly upper-middle-class children. She wanted/needed to put her efforts into helping the poor and needy. This motivation is what brought her (in her wheelchair) to our St. Petersburg Free Clinic to almost beg Butch to allow her to volunteer her services. Had she not wanted so much to work in the clinic, I'm sure that Butch would not have been able to convince her to come and see me.

During that first visit I began treatment with acupuncture, nutritional advice, megavitamin therapy and CranioSacral Therapy. I couldn't do any traditional osteopathic manipulation because to touch her body between the waist and knees with intent to manipulate bone or deep tissue was to make her scream in pain. I couldn't see how this poor lady was living with all this pain. Her blood tests for rheumatoid arthritis were positive.

I set up weekly appointments with her. We soon discovered that acupuncture, when appropriately applied, gave complete relief of pain. In a few weeks we found that one acupuncture needle inserted in the end of her right middle finger for 15 minutes a day controlled her pain well enough so that she could get out of her wheelchair, get away from crutches, and tolerate some more-traditional osteopathic manipulative work. I'm sure that as the pain diminished, the nutritional changes began their effect. In my opinion, motion is necessary for health, so we worked very hard on the re-establishment of movement of the bones, joints and other tissues all the way from her head to her toes.

To make a long story short, Sister Anne was rehabilitated almost completely within a year. She worked ceaselessly at our Free Clinics (there were three of them by now). She became the Free Clinic director as a full-time occupation after obtaining permission from her church authority. Her blood tests for rheumatoid arthritis had returned to normal after 20 years.

Sister Anne and the Upledger family became very good friends. When I left Florida and moved to Michigan in 1975 in order to join the faculty at Michigan State University, Sister Anne and I stayed in close touch with each other. Her condition continued to improve. She didn't need my "doctor" work anymore.

Within a year of our move to Michigan, Sister Anne came to visit us. During this visit she asked my advice about her embarkation upon a program at the University of Florida that would lead her to a degree as a licensed physician's assistant. She wanted to work at the migrant farm labor camps in Florida. I suggested that should she pursue this course, she would always be dependent upon the supervision of a licensed physician to do her work. Why not get her own license as a physician and be independent to do things as she felt they should be done? After some discussion about her age, her lack of premedical requirements, and the difficulties of getting through medical or osteopathic medical school and internship, she finally went out into the woods behind our house for a few hours. She did what deeply spiritual people do, and came back with an "OK, let's try it. What do I do next?"

I arranged an interview with the admissions officer of the College of Osteopathic Medicine at Michigan State University. He was so impressed with Sister Anne that he asked me what we could do to get her to apply there.

She then obtained permission to embark on such a program from her mother house. She completed one year of premedical work in St. Petersburg and then moved in with us in Michigan (East Lansing) to complete her second year of premedical requirements. Next came acceptance into the Osteopathic College and four years of very hard work. After graduation and being awarded her doctor of osteopathic medicine degree, she moved to Detroit for a year of internship. During this year she made an in-depth study of the poverty-stricken and needy areas of the southeastern United States. She settled in Tutweiler, Mississippi, where today she operates a very busy clinic and carries on a tremendous emergency and family medicine practice. All of this from a woman who, in the mid-years of her life, was in a wheelchair, was in constant and great pain, and was contemplating replacement of both her hip joints by surgically inserted mechanical devices.

We talked to Sister/Doctor Anne during the preparation of this manuscript. I asked her what, in her opinion, was the real key to her healing. Without hesitation she replied that it was 80 percent my attitude and intention and 20 percent the mixture of acupuncture, nutrition, CranioSacral Therapy and all the rest.

We therapists should always keep in mind the tremendous power that our intention, attitude and expectation has with the patient and his/her response to treatment. A gloom-and-doom forecast by the healthcare practitioner may well cause the patient to live down to that expectation. The reverse is also true. In Sister Anne's case, we just wouldn't take no for an answer.

Coma Case History

I am fully convinced that the fates give you a great success initially in order to "hook" you into a project. Such has been the case for me with comas. I haven't had much work with true coma patients as yet. I've worked only with a dozen or so thus far in my career, but they have been quite intriguing.

The hook was set the deepest recently by an experience with a coma patient that astonished even me. I was asked to see a 24-year-old girl who had been in a coma for $3^{1}/_{2}$ years since an auto accident. She was a beautiful girl before the accident. She loved life, boyfriends, champagne, dancing, parties and the like. She was the daughter of rather well-to-do Belgian parents.

As I listened to the description of this girl from the mother, I began to feel an intuitive sense about what I should do.

The girl (let's call her Cherie) was lying in the bed in a contracted state. She had one tube in her nose, one in her bladder, and she was wearing a diaper. Her fists were clenched, the right tighter than the left. Her feet were powerfully turned in. Her legs were bent and prevented from crossing only by a pillow placed between her knees. Her eyes were closed. She was unresponsive to my voice and to my pinching on various places on her body.

I gave myself over completely to my intuition. I forced her left hand open enough so that I could slide my fingers into her fist. She reflexively held my fingers tightly in her hand. With my right hand I cradled the back of her head. (I have rather large hands.) I felt the craniosacral rhythm at the back of her head and began working to increase the amplitude of that rhythmical pulse. Then I did something that surprised even me. I began whispering in her ear. I told Cherie that she was beautiful. I told her that if she would only wake up we could drink champagne together and dance all night. We could have a wonderful time together, etc., etc. I have never done anything like this before.

As I gently whispered into her ear, I could feel the amplitude of her craniosacral rhythm increasing and feeling more vital and alive. I continued whispering "sweet nothings" into her ear. When I used certain words her craniosacral rhythm would stop for just an instant. Within a very few minutes she opened her eyes for the first time in 3 1/2 years. She looked at me and squeezed my left hand a little harder as though to tell me that she understood.

I thought that I was being transported to heaven. What a wonderful experience. The mother, the nurse and the mother's friend were all astonished. They were talking and babbling all at once. Joy was palpable in the room.

I treated Cherie daily for seven days. I was teaching a class in Holland at the time, and I brought five students with me for each treatment session after that initial one. By the end of the week Cherie was being hand-fed soft foods. She didn't need the tube through her nose into her stomach anymore. She was holding her head up and moving it around. Her neck was working. She was beginning to gain control of her left hand. She was loosening the spasticity in her right arm and both legs. And she was beginning to move voluntarily, especially her left leg.

Recently I received a letter from Cherie's mother. She told me that Cherie is now talking in a soft voice. You can't imagine what this means to all of us.

Our plan for Cherie is to have our students treat her weekly until her improvement seems to reach a standstill. When and if this occurs I will do some more work with Cherie in order to move her from her plateau back into the improvement mode again. We won't stop until either Cherie is fully recovered or one of us dies. I do hope that my wife will allow me to take Cherie dancing just once when she is able.

Do you see what I mean about getting hooked?

There is room for a lot of research in this area. We are doing some and find it fascinating. We have enough evidence to support the "attitude-effect" concept so that we preach the gospel of "if you have a poor attitude toward a patient, let someone else treat them." We advise therapists that if they have problems in their personal life that they can't leave outside the treatment room door that day, take the day off. The therapist's attitude (be he/she a surgeon, physician, dentist, physical therapist, Rolfer, acupuncturist, CranioSacral Therapist, or anyone else) has much to do with the success of the patient in his/her healing process. With this in mind, therapists should always intention their touch and their attitude in a positive direction. More about this later.

19

Therapeutic Imagery and Dialogue*sm*

When I was in osteopathic medical school, I did several extracurricular things. One was to take a night course in hypnotherapy from a local psychiatrist. He was perhaps a little crazy, but he taught a very good 10-week course. There were eight of us who took his seminar. As I began my practice in Clearwater, Florida, I used the hypnosis to some extent, but soon got too busy with general medicine and surgery to spend the one-on-one time to do hypnosis very often.

Then along came Reta. She was 38 years old, had four children who were all in school, and an engineer husband who sometimes worked and sometimes didn't. He was very abusive to her verbally. Occasionally he physically abused her. Reta was the mainstay of the family; she held it together. She was the executive secretary for a local bank president. She was highly valued and under paid. She ran the president's office and he knew it, but to admit this fact would have been difficult for him. It was partly a pride issue, plus he knew that if he let her know her real value she might very likely be difficult to control; she might even ask for a raise.

Reta was referred to me because she had uncontrollable and unrelenting pain in her head, neck, upper thorax, shoulders, arms and hands. She had less frequent, but episodically severe, low-back and right-sciatic pain. She was referred to me by an orthopedic surgeon who couldn't find anything else to cut on. He had operated on her three times already. He had been unsuccessful in helping her. I had developed some small reputation as a pain controller who used hypnosis, trigger injection, manipulation and whatever else was available. Rumor also had it that I did a pretty fair brand of general medicine and minor surgery. Reta was probably a nuisance to the orthopedist by now, as well as a reminder that he had failed. He knew that I would take the night calls because I was young, eager and rather taken with myself.

Reta had been surgically cut upon and generally punished significantly for most of her life. She had her varicose veins surgically removed. She had a hysterectomy after her fourth obstetrical delivery. All four children had been delivered vaginally with wide episeotomies. She then underwent a repair of the perineum and a bladder suspension, both done before the hysterectomy. She then had her gallbladder removed. This referring orthopedic surgeon had removed discs from between the third and fourth as well as from between the fourth and fifth lumbar vertebrae. These were done on two separate occasions. After this he had unsuccessfully attempted nerve-root decompression in the lower cervical region.

In addition to all this, her children were very demanding of her time and energy. They offered very little respect. I simply listened to her story, examined her body, felt a lot of compassion, and vowed aloud that we would get to the bottom of this problem. Reta and I made a pact that we would work together on this problem until we reached a solution.

I began by using trigger injections according to what I had learned of Dr. Janet Travell's method. Dr. Travell had been John F. Kennedy's back-pain doctor. I had experienced some success with this method when I coupled it with osteopathic manipulation. In Reta's case, I didn't get to first base. She only got worse. In desperation I began to see her at night as my last patient so that I could begin using some hypnosis on her. My intention was to train her in self-hypnosis so that she could learn to relax herself and get more sleep.

She learned to relax to some degree during the early sessions. Suddenly, during one of these sessions, she began to regress rather spontaneously to a very young age. I recognized that she was ready to do something, but I didn't know what. I got the idea that maybe we could use this occasion to find out if there was a reason for the pain that might be emotional rather than physical. This was in 1966, before I knew about acupuncture, CranioSacral Therapy, SomatoEmotional Release, and the like. Under hypnosis I asked her to go back to the time when the reason for the pain was implanted. This was a tedious process because, as she regressed to an infant, she could not talk intelligibly to me. She had to write everything out. I didn't know at the time that I could have requested that an adult-witness part of her go up to the ceiling and describe the scene to me. Instead I suggested that she could retain her ability to write as an adult.

After many questions and a lot of written answers (people write rather slowly under these circumstances), Reta regressed to the age of 2 days. She had been born at home and was lying in a cradle. Her mother and maternal grandmother were there. Her grandmother was admonishing her mother for having another baby at her age. (Mother was 42 years old at the time of Reta's birth.) Reta was the youngest of eight children. Grandma said that "Reta should never have been born; it was too hard on Mother." Grandma also said that Reta would never be healthy. The imposition of guilt and hopelessness upon Reta from this conversation was phenomenal. I shall never forget what Reta wrote when I asked her how she felt about this scene. She wrote, "If I had to be born, if I had to live, at least I can be weak, sick and hurt all my life."

When Reta came out of her regressed hypnotic state, I very gently asked her if she could read what was written on the paper. She could not. She asked me if I could read it, and I pretended that I could not. She accepted this explanation without any question. She wanted to believe me. Three days later we repeated the same regression to the cradle, and she listened again to her grandmother talking to her mother. She wrote me the same statement again about how she felt. This time I was a little wiser. I told her that the pregnancy was not instigated by her. I told her that all had gone well. Her mother had survived the delivery without difficulty. I told her that her grandmother probably meant well, but that her observations were not correct. I wasn't sure that I got through to her because Reta was still the 2-day-old infant when I delivered my speech. Again I let her know, as she was returning to the here and now, that she did not need to comprehend anything that she was not ready for. I was painstakingly careful about imparting this message to her. She could not read her handwritten message.

Four days later, Reta came in again. Hypnotic trance was quickly induced. I asked her to go to the experience whereby she became convinced that she could not be without pain. She went straight to the same cradle scene. She heard her grandmother's words to her mother for the third time. I delivered my lecture again about the pregnancy not being Reta's responsibility and so on. Then I intuitively brought her back to adulthood while still in deep trance. We discussed the situation while in hypnotic trance as an adult. Reta agreed that it was not valid that she should spend her life in pain because of her grandmother's emotional words to her mother. We also agreed that she would be able to handle the insight after she came out of the trance. I brought Reta back to her usual state of conscious awareness. She was able to read her notes this time. She simply asked whether she could have done all this to herself. I replied that it seemed reasonable to me that she could have.

Strange as it seems, that was the end of Reta's pain. She divorced her husband. She quit her job. She started her own real estate company in partnership with a man who eventually became her husband. Reta was an excellent teacher for me. I am forever grateful to her.

Reta's case planted in my mind the early concepts of the potential for the influence of the mind over the body.

A little later in my conventional medical/surgical career (if I was ever conventional), another experience occurred that opened my eyes even further about the interrelationship between mind and body. This occurred when I hospitalized a young lady in her early 20s with an acute problem in the lower right area of the abdomen. The choices were acute appendicitis, rupturing cyst on her right ovary, and/or inflammation of some of the lymph nodes in the tissues near the appendix and/or the ovary. The surgeon I had asked to consult favored the diagnosis of acute appendicitis. All the signs were there except for one of my favorites, which wasn't generally accepted as valid anyway. This sign was pain at the tip of the lowest (12th) rib on the right. I had observed that if this rib tip wasn't painful to the touch, the problem probably would not be appendicitis. The surgeon was quite sure it was appendicitis, and I was not yet self-confident enough to argue with him based on a 12th rib tip that wasn't painful to the touch.

The patient was scheduled for surgery the next morning. I was to serve as first assistant to the surgeon whom I had asked to consult. He was my favorite and most trusted surgeon.

Something possessed me the night before surgery. I went in to see this patient and decided to see if I could hypnotize her. It was easily done. She was partially medicated to relax her and went very quickly into a deep trance. I asked her if there was a physician inside of her who knew what was wrong. Without the slightest hesitation, she said that there was. I asked if I might be privileged to speak and consult with this Inner Physician. She agreed. Her voice changed to a lower register and said, "Hello, I am the Inner Physician." I asked the Inner Physician if she knew what was wrong inside. (It sounded like a feminine voice even though it was lower in pitch than the patient's normal speaking voice.) The Inner Physician answered without hesitation that the problem was a ruptured ovarian cyst. I accepted this answer, thanked the Inner Physician for her help, and instructed the patient to either go deeper into normal sleep or wake up, whichever she preferred. She awoke. I made some small talk and went home.

The next morning while the surgeon and I were scrubbing before entering the operating room, I asked him if he was still convinced that we would find an acute appendicitis. He answered that he was sure. I disagreed mildly and respectfully. I then enticed him to bet me $5. I would take the ovary diagnosis and he would take the appendicitis. We operated. It was an ovarian cyst that had ruptured. The surgery went along uneventfully and, when we were finished, he paid me the $5 he owed me.

After that I used the hypnosis approach to diagnosis on several occasions. The surgeon would not bet me anymore. The Inner Physicians of these patients always gave me correct information. It was amazing. There was actually a part of the nonconscious of each patient that knew precisely what was wrong with them. Later on I discovered that these Inner Physicians also had very valuable information about why the problem was present and about the best method of treatment.

Another personal experience helped to expand my understanding of the use of Therapeutic Imagery and Dialogue. This occurred at a seminar wherein I was the demonstration subject. This was a group primarily composed of psychologists and psychotherapists. The course was being conducted by Marty Rossman, M.D., who has been teaching what he calls "Guided Imagery" for a long time.

Marty finished a lecture and asked for a volunteer from the audience upon whom he could demonstrate the technique of imaging a pain or problem. I volunteered because no one else seemed eager to do so. I had no special agenda that I was aware of when I went to the front of the room, and I didn't really know what to expect.

I sat on a stool across from Marty. He asked me what I would like to get acquainted with. After some thought, I mentioned that I had experienced pain across my low back and into my right sacroiliac off and on for many years. I then remembered first going to an osteopath for this pain when I was 14 years old. Marty asked me if I could look down inside my back and get an image of the pain. I tried, and the image came very easily. The pain was red and shaped like a boomerang. Marty suggested that I ask the boomerang to tell me more about itself. I asked, and the boomerang began to inflate like a beach toy that someone was blowing up. As it inflated, my back pain began to act up. It grew more painful as the boomerang continued to inflate. I asked what was inflating it. The answer that popped into my head was a single word, very definite. That word was ANGER. Then I got the idea that anger was like a boomerang; when you are angry, it comes back at you. When I was angry, my back hurt. My back pain began shortly after the untimely death of my father. I was really angry at God for taking my father away from me.

What I have learned is that no amount of physical treatment or manipulation can take away this back pain when I have it. But I can sit down in a quiet place and introspect about whether I am angry or not and, if so, what about. When I find the anger and resolve it, my back pain automatically goes away. This has been the case since my introduction to the "boomerang" about eight or 10 years ago. It is amazing how often I used to be angry and not be aware of it. After I learned that a back pain meant I was angry, whether I knew it or not, I learned to deal with being angry much more effectively. I have back pain a lot less than I used to. When it does come, I know that it is time to sit down away from everything and discover what I'm angry about. Now I realize that when I'm aware of being angry, my back doesn't hurt. It only hurts when I'm angry and don't know it. Anger can kill you. My back pain tells me when I'm angry so that I can do something about it. I love my back pain. It has probably prolonged my life. It may even have prevented a heart attack. I think my back pain is a message from my Inner Physician.

Now let's look at the concept of Inner Physician, Therapeutic Imagery and Dialogue, and what these things can do to benefit you.

As you may have guessed by now, I have come to believe each and every one of us has an intelligence inside that knows everything about what is going on in our lives. This includes our symptoms and their meanings (if any), our illnesses, our inner conflicts, and the like. My experience supports this belief quite strongly. In fact, the belief is a result of my experience. Some people would explain this in terms of a universal consciousness to which we are all connected. Other people feel that we each have an individual wisdom inside that knows about the body and/or person in which it lives, but not too much about anyone else. Many people believe that they have spirit guides that know everything about them. There are many, many more ideas about these things. What you believe or how you get that belief is strictly up to you.

My belief is that somewhere inside of you is the answer to every question that can be asked about you. My concern, as your healthcare practitioner, is that we make a connection with that part of you that knows the answers, and that those answers can be shared with us and used for the good of the total you.

Since most of what we deal with is health related, unless the patient has another preference, we call this part of their consciousness the Inner Physician. In the use of CranioSacral Therapy we have found that the great majority of patients enter deep states of relaxation during the treatment process. It is in this state of deep relaxation that we can invite the Inner Physician to come and talk to us. I love to meet Inner Physicians. They always have very wise answers to questions about health and life. Once we have made this contact with the Inner Physician, we develop a friendly rapport. I encourage the patient to get a mental image of this Inner Physician, as well as a name by which it would like to be addressed. Within a short time, after assurances have been made that our intentions are honorable and sincere, we can begin to ask questions that are pertinent to the issue at hand. If the Inner Physician doesn't have an answer, you can suggest that he/she call upon a consultant from the nonconscious. Ultimately some part of the patient knows the answer.

When the real Inner Physician appears, the craniosacral rhythm stops. You are on the track of some significant material. So we use the craniosacral rhythm as a significance detector. When it stops, something important is in the patient's mind. Sometimes a patient's nonconscious parts, or Inner Physicians, play tricks on the therapist. They may present answers that are misleading or incorrect. When the material under discussion is not significant, the craniosacral rhythmic activity keeps on going. When this occurs, you know that you are on a wild-goose chase.

Let me show you how this works. A 42-year-old lady came to see me. She had been referred by some friends. I was a sort of desperate last stop. She had suddenly come down with acute glaucoma in both eyes. It was not being successfully controlled by medications. She had lost about 20 percent of her visual field already, and the outlook did not look good because the pressure in her eyes was not coming down although several medications had been tried. She was seeing her ophthalmologist every two weeks. If things continued as they were, she could be virtually blind in a year or so.

She came in for CranioSacral Therapy because she had heard that this type of treatment could help a wide variety of problems. I did some CranioSacral work with her, focusing mostly on the bones of the orbits of the eyes. My intent was to improve fluid drainage from the eyes and the related tissues. (Glaucoma is a disease that is characterized by increased fluid pressure inside the eyeball.) I also directed energy through the eyeballs individually during this first session. The treatment I did had no beneficial effect on the eyeball pressure of either eye.

During the next treatment session, I used CranioSacral Therapy techniques to take her to a very relaxed state. When she seemed to be in deep relaxation, I asked her very quietly if there was a physician inside of her who knew the cause of the glaucoma. Her craniosacral system activity stopped, and she said, "Yes, there is." I asked if that physician inside of her would come forward so that we could get acquainted. Her craniosacral rhythm stopped, but she said nothing. I asked her what was in her mind right at that time. She said that there was only a seagull soaring in circles out over a seashore. I asked if the seagull was her Inner Physician. She said that she didn't know. I asked, "Seagull, are you the Inner Physician?" She said the seagull said "yes." At the same time, the craniosacral rhythm stopped, so I knew that the seagull was the image in which the Inner Physician had chosen to present. Inner Physicians are like magicians. They can come forward in any form that they choose. I think they like to have fun with us. Sometimes I think they like to fool or joke with us to see if we are open-minded and adept enough to work with them.

The seagull sat on the beach in front of the patient. I asked the patient to very politely ask by what name the Inner Physician would like to be known. The answer was "Mermaid." I then introduced myself to Mermaid as John. I said that I was trying to help the patient with her glaucoma. I assured Mermaid that I was sincere in my desire to help, and that I would be most grateful for any help that she could give us with this glaucoma problem. Mermaid said that there were things that the patient did not want to see, so she was going to make herself blind. When this was done, she would not have to see things that she didn't want to see. I suggested to Mermaid that, although the patient might not physically see things by being blind, she would still perceive what was happening and be affected by these events. Mermaid agreed and suggested that we needed to convince the patient that going blind was not going to keep her from knowing what was going on. I asked Mermaid if she would present to us, in the form of a memory, one of the things that the patient did not want to see. I then felt the craniosacral system stop its rhythmical activity. I asked the patient what was in her mind right then. She said that she was thinking about her first husband. He was tall, handsome, charming, and unfaithful to her. She went a long time without seeing the signs of his womanizing. She

119

finally divorced him after she stopped denying his adulterous behavior to herself. The patient was now remarried and did not want to "see" anything that her second husband might do that was suggestive of him being unfaithful, so she would make herself blind.

I asked Mermaid if that was all there was to the glaucoma. Mermaid said, "No, but that was enough for the present." The patient's eyeball pressure stayed the same. It did not elevate further, but it did not decrease either.

I saw this patient in another week. Using CranioSacral Therapy she went into a relaxed state similar to the week before. I asked her to invite Mermaid to join us, if she would like, for further conversation about the glaucoma. The patient's craniosacral rhythm stopped abruptly. The patient said nothing. I asked what images she might be seeing right then. The patient responded that she was at the seashore again and there was a swimmer way off in the distance out in the ocean. I asked if the swimmer was Mermaid. The answer was "yes." I said, "Hello, Mermaid," and visualized the swimmer way out in the water. In my own image, I waved at the swimmer and she waved back. I frequently try to image the same thing the patient images. Usually we see the same things. In this instance, I asked the patient if the swimmer waved, and she said "yes." Now I knew that we were all tuned-in to the same wavelength. I asked Mermaid if she would please show us more of the reason why the patient was losing her vision. There was no answer. The patient began sharing, however, that she saw a black car parked off the road at the beach. She was 4 years old. She and her 2-year-old sister were pounding on the door of the car asking to be let in. Her mother's voice was heard from inside telling her and her sister to go back out on the beach and play for a while longer. It was cold, and the car windows were steamed up so that she couldn't see in, and the car door was locked so that she couldn't open the door.

Her mother and a strange man had taken them all to the seashore in this car. The patient and her sister were told to go out to the beach and play in the sand. They did for a while, but it got cold and no one else was at the seashore that day. The little girls wanted to get back into the car but were denied entry because mother and the man apparently wanted to be alone for a while longer. The patient was old enough now to understand that the man was her mother's lover. She didn't know it, though, when she was 4 years old. The patient's father was an officer in the merchant marine. He was frequently gone for weeks at a time. Her mother had several men friends. The patient didn't want to see that her mother, whom she loved dearly, was unfaithful to her father, whom she also loved dearly. She would rather go blind than see this.

Now that the patient understood the problem and had become acquainted with Mermaid, she did not have to go blind in order to hide from the truth. The patient and Mermaid agreed to have meetings every morning after that so they could talk and get to know each other better.

The ophthalmologist told this patient that the pressure in her eyeballs was almost normal. He also said that there must be some mistake because her visual field loss had improved, yet everyone knows that this improvement would be impossible; there must have been some mistake in the previous tests. The patient reports that she feels good now. She continued to meet and talk with her imaginary friend and Inner Physician, Mermaid, every day. She knows that if she tells her friends about this experience, they will think she is crazy. So she keeps our secret. She hasn't even told her new husband what happened. It is kind of crazy, but then what's a little craziness if it cures glaucoma and prevents blindness?

This is another fine example of the power of mind over body, as well as the power of integrating the processes of CranioSacral Therapy with Therapeutic Imagery and Dialogue.

20

The Bottom Line

The bottom line is the result. We find that when we integrate CranioSacral Therapy, Tissue Memory, Energy Cyst Release, SomatoEmotional Release and Therapeutic Imagery and Dialogue with whatever else we have in our bag of therapeutic tricks, we get results. There are now a rather large number of therapists from a wide variety of healthcare disciplines who integrate all of these therapeutic approaches. We have over a thousand of them who have completed our seminars up to the advanced level, and a few hundred who have completed the advanced seminars. These are all dedicated therapists who have learned to use the treatment methods mentioned above in order to obtain good results for their patients. We all network and work together. There is very little jealousy among us. The political boundaries between professions are being shattered. Chiropractors are talking to medical doctors; osteopaths are talking to dentists.

The Supreme Court of Colorado recently gave two rulings that CranioSacral Therapy could be used by dentists to work below the neck because the craniosacral system affects the teeth and the occlusion. These opinions mean that a dentist in Colorado can now legally manipulate your tailbone to fix your temporomandibular joints because the craniosacral system ends in your tail. Other dentists who have completed our advanced seminars have gone to massage school in order to get licensed to legally work with the whole body. The teeth are part of the whole body; they don't exist in isolation.

The Board of Professional Licensure in Florida accepted our opinion that massage therapists can do CranioSacral Therapy. In fact, some of our better CranioSacral Therapy teachers are licensed massage therapists.

The people who do this kind of work are dedicated to their patients and clients above and beyond any loyalty to a specific profession and through any political boundaries. After all, what's more important, the politics or the therapeutic result? Even politicians recognize that the result is the most important thing when they are hurting.

No matter what your therapist's previous training, be it physical therapy, massage therapy, medicine, chiropractic, nursing, occupational therapy or osteopathy, he or she can learn to use the craniosacral approach and its progeny to get good therapeutic results.

21

Who Can Do This Work?

As you may have guessed, I have been rather severely criticized by some of my colleagues for teaching health-enhancing techniques to non-physicians. The feeling is that these people are simply not qualified to do the work.

Please let me explain how this all came about. In 1976 I was preparing to do some CranioSacral Therapy research on learning-disabled children in the Michigan public school system. During a casual conversation, one of the county supervisors of special education made the comment that he estimated that one in 20 children enrolled in the public schools of the state had some sort of brain function problem. He was including seizures, autism, learning disabilities, concentration problems, retardation, speech problems, and so on. I almost fell off my chair. My feeling was that 50 percent of brain dysfunction problems could be helped by Cranio-Sacral Therapy. This meant that 5 percent of all the school children needed to be evaluated, and probably 2 to 3 percent would need definitive CranioSacral Therapy. Who would do all this work? At that time there were about a half-dozen osteopathic physicians in Michigan who could capably evaluate and treat these children. Neither the evaluation process nor the treatment process could be mass-produced. Each required a minimum of 20 minutes of one-on-one, hands-on time with each child. The interest in learning to do Cranio-Sacral Therapy was not high amongst my physician colleagues. Nor was it high amongst the allopathic and osteopathic medical students we were teaching at the University. The percentage of students interested in pursuing this kind of work was probably 10 percent or less.

As far as I was concerned, every month that passed for a learning-disabled child where he or she went untreated and continued on in school feeling inferior and inadequate was a month of deepening emotional trauma. We needed another way to make craniosacral system evaluation and treatment available to these needy children.

As luck would have it, one of the therapists at a local school for multiply handicapped children knew Olivier, the Belgian child with cerebral palsy whom I described earlier in this book. This therapist had seen Olivier when he was hemiplegic, and later on when he was walking. The therapist knew the effect of CranioSacral Therapy on Olivier. I approached this school with the idea of teaching a course in craniosacral system evaluation to their staff. My idea was to have the evaluation done by non-physicians. Those children who were then identified as good candidates for CranioSacral Therapy would be referred to me for treatment. The enthusiasm of the therapist who had seen Olivier before and after CranioSacral Therapy furnished about 80 percent of the energy required to obtain approval for such a course.

I then went to the dean of my college. I described my plight about the one in 20 children needing evaluations. I obtained his permission to teach a night course for non-physicians at the school for multiply handicapped children. From there I went to the university curriculum office and we obtained post-graduate credit from Michigan State University for all those enrollees who had previous degrees in various fields.

The enrollment in this first one-semester course was about 20 students. There were physical therapists, occupational therapists, registered nurses, school psychologists and a couple of special education teachers. The non-physician students learned the craniosacral system evaluation techniques exceedingly well, and there was a strong demand for a second semester of the course continuation. I could not handle the number of candidates for CranioSacral Therapy whom they identified and referred to me for treatment.

Soon I began to teach them some of the treatment techniques I used when they accompanied the referred child to our clinic. It did not take long for me to realize that being a physician of any kind was not requisite to becoming proficient in craniosacral system evaluation and treatment. Soon I was teaching the night courses in craniosacral system evaluation and treatment sponsored by Michigan State University to any enrollee who had the credentials to work with a child in any diagnostic or therapeutic way.

I began to know that the requirements to do good Cranio-Sacral Therapy were dedication, compassion, sensitivity, and the like. The requisites were not organic chemistry, neurology, materia medica, and other science courses.

I developed what we call a 10-Step Protocol. This is a series of 10 hands-on steps that, if done with reasonable correctness, will help a patient's craniosacral system to work better whether you, as therapist, know what you are doing or not. If you use your hands gently, and don't try to force anything, you can't do any damage.

Soon we were teaching these 10-Step Protocol techniques to the parents of brain-dysfunctioning children so that they could continue their child's treatment independent of our clinic. We did this initially so that they did not have to structure their lives to provide proximity to a CranioSacral Therapist. They could be free. These kinds of cases could return to our clinic two to three times a year for re-evaluation, and the child could get the benefit of uninterrupted CranioSacral Therapy from the parents.

Then we began to realize that this approach of teaching the parents to treat the child regularly (usually on a daily basis) began to bring the family together. It enhanced the feeling of self-worth of the parents when they could do something for their child.

We saw that, in many cases, the mother had been taking over the care of the handicapped child. The father felt left out and useless. We began to develop treatment techniques that required mother and father to work on the child at the same time. More often than not, these couples began to solidify their marriage again. Father was not out in the cold, he was in the loop. He felt useful and necessary. This was good therapy for all concerned.

Next we began to teach father to use simple CranioSacral Therapy techniques on mother when she got a headache. It helped. She felt that he cared. He felt useful. Frustration levels dropped because self-worth and caring levels went up. I'm sure a lot of relationships have been healed because the touch required to do the CranioSacral Therapy techniques is well-intentioned and loving. Touch communicates feeling.

Now we teach one-day seminars around the country called ShareCare sm. We teach a few basic CranioSacral Therapy techniques that have general helping effects. They are not dangerous. Any side effects that occur from improper use are temporary and cause only mild discomfort; no damage is done. We teach the direction of healing energy so that you can help yourself and your friends with aches and pains. If something serious is wrong, the pain may leave, but it will come back soon. If it comes back four or five times, you need a diagnosis by a physician. We introduce you to your Inner Physician. We help you get acquainted, and hope that we can create a setting so that you can converse with your Inner Physician on a daily basis. Yes, you will be talking to yourself, but in so doing you will get to know yourself better. You don't have to tell anyone where you are getting your information.

22

The Anatomy of the Craniosacral System

Where do we find trouble in the craniosacral system? Anything that interferes with the ability of the dura mater membrane to accommodate the rhythmically fluctuating fluid pressures and volumes is a potential trouble source. These membranes form a waterproof bag inside your body. I think of this bag and its contents as forming a hydraulic system in your body. It functions as your "core." Let's look at the anatomy of that dura mater membrane bag and all of its attachments.

If it were taken out of your body, this membrane bag that is so essential to the craniosacral system would look somewhat like a pollywog or tadpole. The head portion of this pollywog would be enclosed in your skull. It attaches to the inside of the skull bones and actually becomes the lining of that part of your skull that we call the cranial vault. The cranial vault sits above the roof of your mouth and over the top of your neck. As the waterproof lining of your skull or cranial vault, this dura mater membrane prevents the fluid that is inside from leaking out. Sometimes we see skull injuries or other problems that create tears or holes in this dura mater layer of the meningeal membrane. When this happens, the fluid of the craniosacral system, called the cerebrospinal fluid, may leak out. Most often I have seen it coming from the nose. Only twice have I seen it leaking from an ear. When a leak occurs,

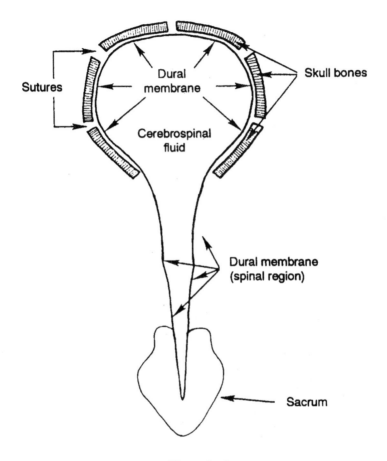

Illustration 8
Semi-closed hydraulic system of the
cerebrospinal fluid and dural membrane

there is a significant opening for infection. Also, the leak results in an increased rate of outflow of fluid from the hydraulic (craniosacral) system. In order to maintain the normal, constant fluid volume inside the hydraulic system, the fluid input or production must be increased when there is a leak. If the fluid production system can handle the increased demand, we usually don't see any problem. On the other hand, if the leak is too big for the production system to accommodate, we get a chronic reduction of fluid volume and, therefore, a reduction in the amplitude of the rhythmical pressure fluctuation in the craniosacral system.

Usually this person suffers from a multitude of symptoms, many of which may be erroneously ascribed to other causes. The symptom or complaint list includes such things as chronic fatigue, recurrent dull headaches, generalized aches and pains all over the body (focusing mostly on the more vulnerable or previously injured areas), inability to concentrate, and a general lack of energy so that self-starting on a project is very difficult. It requires a great deal of self-discipline and determination to go on with life. Not quite as consistently we also see a significant reduction of resistance to infections. That is, every time someone within a hundred yards sneezes, this person catches a cold. We may also see a hormonal imbalance that manifests as low thyroid function, low blood sugar (hypoglycemia) and/or menstrual problems. Such are the possibilities when there is a significant leak in our dura mater membrane bag and the craniosacral hydraulic system is unable to keep up with the deficit.

Nature has created a beautiful design in this system. As I said before, within your skull or cranial vault the dura mater membrane forms the waterproof lining. At the base of your skull, where the skull joins your neck, is an opening. This opening is somewhat oval in shape, about $1^1/_2$ to 2 inches

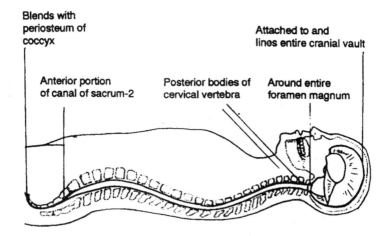

Blends with
periosteum of
coccyx

Attached to and
lines entire cranial vault

Anterior portion
of canal of sacrum-2

Posterior bodies of
cervical vertebra

Around entire
foramen magnum

Illustration 9
Points of attachment of dura (detail)

across, and is located so that it is equally divided by the front-to-back midline of your body. This opening has been named the foramen magnum. In Latin, foramen means "opening" and magnum means "great." It is clear how this great opening in the base of your skull got its name. It is this great opening that affords passage of the spinal cord out of the skull and into the spinal canal. This is where the tail of our polly-wog begins. There is a very firm attachment of the dura mater membrane around this great opening in the base of the skull. Then the dura mater membrane forms a rather long, roughly cylindrical tube (the tail of the pollywog) that drops through the spinal canal as though it were suspended from its ring of attachment around the great opening (foramen magnum) in the base of the skull. So now we have the vertebral column forming a spinal canal through which the tube of dura mater membrane passes. Inside this tube of dura mater membrane is the arachnoid membrane and the pia mater membrane of which I spoke earlier. We have tubes within tubes within which the very delicate spinal cord passes from your head (where it is an extension of your brain) all the way down to your low back.

The outermost tube, which is formed by the vertebrae of the spine, is made up of bone, tough ligaments and other connective-type tissues. The attachments of the outermost layer of the membrane tubes (the dura mater) inside the bony spinal canal are minimal. There are two attachments of the front side (anterior) of this dura mater membrane tube to the upper vertebrae of the neck. And there are attachments of the same dura mater membrane way down in the low back. These attachments are to the front side (anterior) of the triangular bone that fits between the pelvic bones. The triangular bone is called the sacrum. This sacrum has in it a continuation of the spinal canal that opens to its back side about three-fourths of

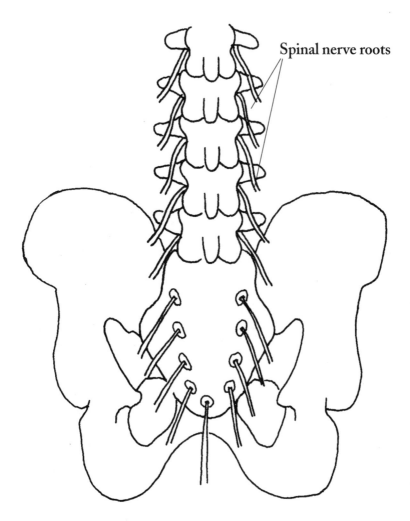

Illustration 10
Back (posterior) view of sacrum and lower spinal vertebra
showing exit of spinal nerve roots from within spinal canal

the way down. The dura mater membrane has some attachment to the sacrum inside this canal. Then it comes out the opening in the lower back side of the sacrum and attaches to the tailbone, named the coccyx.

You may be aware that as the spinal cord passes through the spinal canal, it has nerve roots that pass between each two vertebrae all the way from the top of the neck to the low back. There are 24 vertebrae stacked up that form the spinal column between the sacrum at the lower end and the skull on top. Also, the sacrum has little holes in its canal that afford passage for the spinal cord nerve roots to get out before the tail end of the membrane passes through the lower opening of the spinal canal, which is formed in the sacrum.

These nerve roots branch off from the spinal cord and extend laterally both left and right between all of these vertebrae and through the holes (foramena) in the sacrum. The wonderfully designed membrane system follows each of these nerve roots out to the left and to the right for a couple of centimeters as they (the nerve roots) go out into the body and perform all the services for you that nerves do. After following each nerve root this short distance, the dura mater membrane (which as you recall is the outermost layer of the membranes) makes a watertight seal so that the cerebrospinal fluid is kept inside the craniosacral system. These membrane sleeves are not so tight that they prevent movement of the dura mater membrane within the spinal canal.

You should also know that the cerebrospinal fluid inside the dura mater membrane provides a lubricant between the three layers of membrane within the spinal canal. There is also a lubricating fluid on the outside of the dura mater membrane between it and the bones that form the spinal canal. This fluid lubrication allows the membranes to glide in relationship to one another and in relationship to the vertebrae as we go

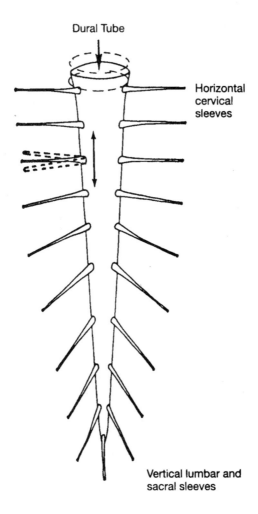

Illustration 11
Mechanics of dural sleeves, which allow up and down
movement of dural tube within the spinal canal

about our normal activities that involve bending and twisting our bodies. If the membranes lose some of their freedom to glide freely, we hurt like crazy and can't move our backs.

One of the most seriously debilitating problems of impaired membrane glide is called "arachnoiditis." This is an inflammation of the middle membrane layer (arachnoid membrane) of the meninges. When the inflammation is present, you are in absolute agony. You can't find a position of relief from the pain, nor can you find a drug sufficiently strong to help much—short of one that knocks you out. Frequently, after the inflammation has died down, there are adhesions that develop and prevent the free gliding of these membranes in relation to each other. So you continue to hurt like crazy, but you may be able to find one or two positions that feel fairly comfortable. You just don't move because it hurts too much. We have found that by using your skull bones, your upper neck vertebrae, and your sacrum and coccyx (bones at the lower end of your spine), we can help this condition a great deal. Using these bones as naturally provided handles on the dura mater membrane, we gently start moving the membrane system up and down in the spinal canal in order to reinstitute the circulation of the fluid between the membrane layers and to break up the cohesion and/or adhesion between membrane layers. The pain usually gets worse as we are going through the treatment process because, at first, we are encouraging raw, non-lubricated membrane layers to rub against each other, and we may be separating adhesions. This sort of feels like putting sandpaper in one of your joints. But the end result is relief of pain and a high percentage of restoration of function to your body.

Other causes for compromise of the free-gliding motion of the spinal canal in relation to the dura mater membrane, and the membrane layers in relation to each other, may include adhesions following spinal cord or meningeal surgery, the injection of dye into the spinal canal for myelogram studies when a ruptured disc is suspected, the placement of a needle into the spinal canal when doing a spinal tap, and so on. Anything that represents an invasion of privacy to the spinal canal and its enclosed membrane system can result in a compromise of the mobility of the meningeal membranes.

As an aside, I share with you an experience of mine that opened the doors to the resolution of a lot of headache problems. During our work at Michigan State University researching the craniosacral system and its evaluation and treatment, we were measuring the movement of the skull bones of live, but anesthetized, monkeys. We could see the skull-bone movement very well and were recording it. During this work I got the idea that we could test whether or not we were dealing with a single and continuous hydraulic system from the skull all the way to the tailbone. We knew that the dura mater membrane was continuous from the top of the head to the tailbone, but there was that tight attachment at the foramen magnum (great opening) in the base of the skull. Did we have a boundary here that might give us two functionally separate hydraulic systems? If so, one system would be above the foramen magnum and the second below it in the spinal canal.

We had our monitoring devices on two bones (parietals) on the top of the monkey's skull. These devices were mounted directly on the skull bones through very small incisions, one on each side of the monkey's head. All I had to do to test the question of whether there were one or two hydraulic systems was to apply a very slight pressure on the monkey's tailbone using the tip of my little finger. Within an instant, the movement of the monkey's skull bones was stopped by my pressure on his tailbone. The pressure applied by my finger was just

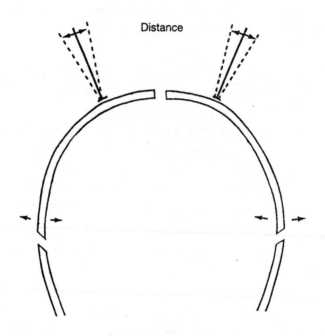

Illustration 12
Experimental setup that demonstrates
movement of monkey skull bones

enough to overcome the power of the fluid production going into the monkey's craniosacral system. The monkey was in a special anesthesia chair designed to keep him in a sitting position. My fingertip pushed up on his tailbone with about enough force to pick up half an ounce before the movement of the skull bones stopped. I found that I could stop and start his skull-bone motion at will by pushing lightly on his tailbone.

Then I got the idea that if you fell on your tailbone, bent it forward, and it stayed there, this situation might place extra tension on the dura mater membrane system in the spinal canal. This increased mechanical membrane tension, along with the resultant compromise in the workings of the hydraulics of the craniosacral system, could cause headaches. Now who would believe that a fall on your tailbone could cause headaches for years afterwards? I tried the idea out on several headache patients. When I found a tailbone that was pushed forward and was able to reposition it back to normal, more than half of the headaches disappeared right there on the spot. Then, to prove the cause and effect relationship, I would bring the headache back by pushing the tailbone forward again. Usually I had to push the tailbone forward and pull it back to normal several times, causing the headache to come and go in synchrony with the tailbone position, in order to demonstrate to the patient that the headache was coming from the other end. After they were convinced of the head-tail relationship, they usually remembered a fall on the tailbone that preceded the onset of the headaches by months or even years. Why do the headaches wait so long to come after the fall? I suspect that is because, for a while, your body can adapt to adversity, but after it tires and loses its adaptability you get symptoms.

23

How the Craniosacral System Evaluation and Treatment Are Carried Out

Now let's look at the ways we can get through to this dura mater membrane that forms the watertight barrier/boundary for the hydraulic system inside of us. We named it the craniosacral system because much of our access to the system is through the bones of the cranium, the upper neck, and the sacrum and coccyx (low back and tailbone).

The quantity or volume of cerebrospinal fluid inside the watertight dura mater membrane bag increases and decreases rhythmically at a rate of about 10 cycles per minute. This rise and fall in fluid volume must be accommodated by the system so that an inordinate amount of hydraulic pressure is not transmitted to its contents, most importantly the brain and spinal cord. These organs reside within our hydraulic system. The brain and spinal cord are not only extremely delicate structures whose functions can be distorted by abnormal pressure changes, they are also very sensitive to chemical changes within their surroundings. Unfavorable chemical changes, including hyperacidity of the cerebrospinal fluid, can result from fluid pressures that are outside the normal range. Increased or abnormal fluid pressures may interfere with the normal delivery of nutrient substances and the removal of waste products. In addition, the brain and spinal cord rely to a great extent upon the generation and delivery of electricity to do their work. Pressure changes can and do impair proper current conduction as well as voltage production and capacitance storage.

With these facts in mind, the question becomes: How does this watertight dura mater membrane bag accommodate the rhythmical fluid pressure changes?

For starters, the membrane inside the spinal canal has reasonable freedom to move up and down within the spinal canal. My own observations during surgical procedures indicate that most of the time these dura mater membrane tubes can glide about one or two centimeters vertically within the spinal canal.

At least this is true in the lumbar region, where most of my observations have been made. The lumbar region is that part of the spine below the rib cage that extends to the sacrum. The sacrum is that triangular bone that fits between the pelvic bones (the ilia) in the back. Some of the craniosacral system's accommodation to fluid pressure changes occurs within the spinal canal. Remember, when I stopped the monkey's sacrum from moving using my finger, the bones of his skull stopped moving with the craniosacral rhythm. This observation illustrates and confirms the unity or oneness of the hydraulic system from the top of the head to the tailbone. It also demonstrates that the fluid pressure within the hydraulic craniosacral system rises enough to stop the movement of the skull bones when you immobilize the lower end (sacral end) of the system. The head end of the system was probably unable to relax between the fluid-filling phases of the craniosacral system. Clearly, part of the accommodation is done by the tail end of the dura mater membrane tube within the spinal canal. This tube has the sacrum and tailbone as its bony handles at the lower end. We have learned how to use these handles in working with the craniosacral system in both the evaluative process and in corrective treatment.

What about the head end of this system? You read about the movement of skull bones in some of my previous descriptions. We watched monkey skull bones move. We feel human skull bones move with our hands. I was taught in osteopathic medical school that by the time we reach puberty (at the very latest), all the bones of the skull are fused solidly together. It is as though we have one solid bone on top of our necks, except for our lower jaws (which continue to move) and the tiny bones in our middle-ear cavities (which vibrate and move in response to various sounds). In other words, at my present age, my head should essentially be solid like a coconut shell with my brain inside of it. This simply is not so. Our research at Michigan State University (1975-1982) did indeed prove beyond any doubt that skull bones continue to move throughout normal life. This movement is much easier to visualize in babies. Many of you are parents or have had the opportunity to hold tiny babies. I'm sure you remember the "soft spots" on the babies' heads. These soft spots are more correctly called fontanelles. Actually these fontanelles are places where the skull bones have not yet expanded to make the hard covering of bone that protects the baby's brain. The dura mater membrane, with its enclosed cerebrospinal fluid, is what you feel beneath the skin if you gently rest your finger on one of these soft spots in the baby's head. It's kind of an eerie and scary feeling to sense that you are so close to an infant's brain.

The brain was first covered by this dura mater membrane during development inside the uterus. Then the membrane began to grow bone on the outer surface between itself and the tissues of the scalp. The bone growth began in very specifically located growth centers on the dura mater

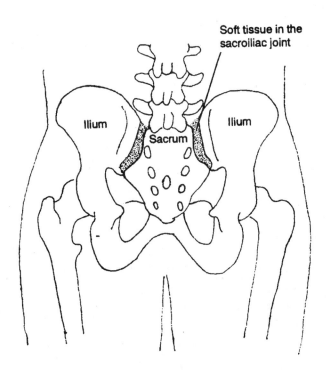

Illustration 13
Back (posterior) view of sacrum between the ilia

membrane. A system of skull bones gradually developed that provided a complete bony protective covering for the brain. The soft spots that you feel in the baby's head disappear over the early weeks and months of infant development. But the bones do not fuse solidly together as we were taught in anatomy class. Some American anatomists recognize this fact today. The edges of the bones of the skull come close together and even abut each other, but throughout life, under normal conditions, a little movement continues to accommodate the rhythmical rise and fall of fluid volume and pressure inside the craniosacral hydraulic system.

The places where the edges of these skull bones come together are actually very specialized joints. These joints between the skull bones have been called sutures. The sutures are of several different designs. The design of the suture tells you what kind of movement it performs. One of the very important sutures is called the sagittal suture. It is where the two parietal bones of your skull meet each other. The suture between these two bones runs in a front-to-back direction over the top of your head. It runs on the midline from about four to six inches above your brow line to about three to four inches up from your hairline in the back. This suture allows for a widening and narrowing of your head that helps to accommodate the fluid volume changes on the inside. The suture is shaped like fingers interdigitating with each other. This design allows for a widening and narrowing movement between the two bones, but it prevents a shearing movement which would occur if one of the parietal bones tried to move forward and the other backward at the same time. This suture design and the movement it allows between the two parietal bones is very similar to the expansion joints that you see in bridges, roads, buildings, etc., that allow for the changes in size produced by the variations in temperature of the air, sunshine, ice accumulation, and so on.

Our studies have shown that, under normal conditions, all of the bones of the skull move rhythmically to accommodate the changing fluid volumes inside the dura mater membrane bag which forms our hydraulic craniosacral system. We have observed that injuries and some diseases may cause a loss of this normal movement of the skull bones. We have seen that we can actually change the distance across the roof of your mouth, the width of your head, in some cases the protrusion of your ears, and sometimes the level of your cheek bones by the use of the techniques we have developed to manipulate and correct "stuckness" of the various bones of the skull.

Since the dura mater membrane is the lining of the skull (cranial vault) and is firmly attached to the inner surface of these skull bones, we can use these bones as handles on the dura mater membrane to produce therapeutic change in the membrane's tensions and in the function of the craniosacral system, per se.

At this juncture I would not be at all surprised if you thought it rather presumptuous of me to assume that you will believe me when I say that skull bones continue to move throughout life under normal conditions. You may think of me as an outrageous egomaniac when I ask you to believe me as I refute the classical teachings of anatomists, which are based on beliefs that began hundreds of years ago. Allow me to help you understand why I'm saying these things about skull bones and fluid pressure.

Let's begin with: Why haven't neurosurgeons/brain surgeons seen the phenomenon that I saw when we operated on Delbert's neck? First of all, most brain surgery begins with a couple of holes being drilled in the patient's head. Since the inner lining of the skull bones is provided by our watertight dura mater membrane, and this membrane must be intact to offer the boundary for the craniosacral hydraulic system to work, the drilled holes immediately destroy the intactness of the hydraulic system. There is no longer a contained fluid pressure that can rise and fall for the surgeon and his/her assistants and nurses to look at. You may recall that one of the goals during our operation on Delbert was to avoid cutting or nicking the dura mater membrane so that we did not open an avenue of infection that could result in meningitis. My personal attention was definitely drawn to the dura mater membrane movement because it was my job to hold it still. I spent at least 45 memorable moments of my life becoming acquainted with this membrane's movements. I learned by demonstration how persistent and rhythmical were its movements. Even in cases where the membrane's intactness is preserved so that the craniosacral system's function continues, it is not highly probable that those involved in the surgery would necessarily notice this membrane moving. Emotional tension is high during an operation, and the attention is highly focused on certain specifics.

Another question is: Why does classical anatomy teach that sutures are fused and immovable by the time we reach early adulthood? I suspect that the answer to this question is simple: Long ago it seemed that way. There was really very little reason to challenge the idea of fusion between skull-bone edges. The motions are very small, on the order of one- or two-sixteenths of an inch. These movements are easy to stop with a little pressure, and are very difficult to see with the human eye. They are much easier to feel with your hands. Now let me tell you what we discovered during our research. First of all, when we studied bone and suture specimens (remember, a suture is the name given to most skull joints) from the anatomy laboratory, it did indeed look like the sutures were fused. Then we got the bright idea that it might be different if we studied little pieces of suture taken from living people at the time of brain surgery. These specimens (from living people) were frozen. They were not treated with preservative chemicals. They were all studied within 12 hours of the time of surgery. What a difference that made. The anatomy laboratory sutures came from skulls that had been preserved in formaldehyde. We studied them months to years after death. The fresh sutures were full of elastic and collagen tissue, nerves and blood vessels. They were very much alive and would most certainly act as a joint allowing a degree of motion between the two skull-bone edges. The old sutures from the anatomy laboratory had lost the distinctiveness of these elastic tissues, nerves and blood vessels. These tissues and structures had all deteriorated so that it looked like one big calcified mess. It was no wonder anatomists did not consider skull sutures as moveable joints.

There is another experience that I would like to share with you regarding the movement of sutures (skull-bone joints). I was invited to Israel during the summer of 1978 as a visiting professor. I went to continue some of my research with Dr. Karni, a biophysicist who had been at Michigan State University the preceding three years. During this stay in Israel I was invited to give a presentation to the hospital staff in Haifa. The topic to be considered was CranioSacral Therapy and its efficacy with learning-disabled children. I was a little nervous because this was such a new and rather revolutionary concept. I expected very sharp and penetrating questions from the audience of physicians and scientists. I presented my case for the ongoing movement of skull bones, one in relationship to the other. I gave slide projections of microscopic views of sutures and so on, ad nauseam.

I did not get much response. Not a single question came from the audience. I thought that I must not have been understood. I began to reiterate this part of my lecture. A friend, Dr. Gidron, who had arranged the presentation, saw my confusion. He very gently interrupted me and suggested that it might be time for a coffee break before I went on to the next topic. I acquiesced. He took me to the hospital library where he located an anatomy book by Professor Guiseppe Sperino published in 1920. He asked me if I could read Italian. I could not. He then translated words from this old anatomy book that told me that in 1920 Professor Sperino stated that skull bones continue to move one in relationship to the other throughout life except under abnormal and/or pathological conditions. I had been telling these fine doctors and scientists something they already knew and took for granted. What a lesson—we had reinvented the wheel back in Michigan. Further investigation showed that the Italian anatomists had decided many years ago that cranial sutures (joints) allow motion between skull bones throughout life. The British anatomists had assumed that cranial bones fuse together by early adulthood and that skull bones don't or can't move in relation to each other after that time. We Americans learned most of our anatomy from the British teachers. These Israeli doctors and scientists had studied mostly from the Italian school. Apparently the British-Italian communication line has been flawed. This is a very valuable lesson to keep in mind when you are struggling to find the truth.

I began this section by asking what we could use to evaluate and correct the function of the craniosacral hydraulic system. The basic answer is now with us: Initially we use the bones to which the dura mater membrane attaches in order to work with the craniosacral hydraulic system.

24

Other Areas of Application for CranioSacral Therapy

CranioSacral Therapy is designed to be used in conjunction with other forms of treatment. It is up to the clinical judgment of the therapist to decide appropriate use in each individual case. It is most often a complement to other forms of treatment—not an alternative.

A word about training for laypersons. The ShareCare program is a one-day, hands-on workshop specifically designed to provide techniques for home care. The workshops are offered by The Upledger Institute and are taught by local Cranio-Sacral Therapy practitioners. The program is offered in the United States, Canada, Europe, New Zealand and Japan.

Acute Systemic Infectious Conditions
The stillpoint technique (CV-4) taught in the ShareCare workshop is extremely valuable to help reduce fevers and to help sufferers pass through the crisis phase of infectious illnesses including measles, chicken pox, influenza, and the like. Usually the stillpoint is repeated two to three times in succession. The fever should drop within an hour after treatment. The fever usually does not return. This would indicate a change or reversal in the illness process. If the fever does rise again, repeat the stillpoint procedure. The CV-4 affects the autonomic nervous system and enhances fluid motion. Used

along with conventional treatment and supportive measures, the CV-4 will often hasten the recovery process.

Localized Infections, Sprains, Strains, Bumps and Bruises
For centuries children have asked their mothers to "make my ouchie better." We have seen that dramatic effects can be realized with a very refined version of what mothers instinctively do. We use the "direction of energy" technique. (This is also taught in the ShareCare workshop.)

Basically, the direction of energy technique is a very simple one. Place one hand on the side of the body part opposite from the bruise, cut, boil, abscess, sprain, strain, infection or bump. Point the fingers of this hand at the problem so that they direct energy at it. These fingers (one, two or three of them) will usually be at approximate right angles to the skin surface they are touching. Now make a cup of your other hand over the problem so that your hand edges are touching around the problem, but not directly on it. Imagine a force traveling from the first hand to the second. The injured area will begin to pulsate as the energy travels from one hand to the other. After a few minutes the pulsations will diminish and the area will soften and start to feel better. The process is repeated two to three times daily until the symptoms feel better and involved tissue looks better. We think of this process as sending reinforcements that strengthen natural body defenses and healing processes.

The direction of energy technique is also used quite effectively in conjunction with tissue-tension balancing techniques for acute sprains and strains. The body part moves back through the positional pattern of the injury to the point of release. It is like watching a movie in reverse. At the position where the injury release can occur, the craniosacral rhythm stops and the tissues soften as the energy pattern of the injury dissipates. The craniosacral rhythm then starts again and returns to normal.

The craniosacral rhythm may also be evaluated over the entire body in order to discover the existence of other less-obvious injury sites that may be contributing to the obvious sprain or strain. Symptoms do not always occur at the site of underlying problems. If the sprain or strain does not clear up quickly with the direction of energy techniques, you may need x-rays and further evaluation by a physician.

Chronic Pain Syndrome
Chronic pain problems respond well to the combination of direction of energy and the other craniosacral and related techniques that have been previously discussed. We often combine the craniosacral approach with Energy Cyst Release, SomatoEmotional Release, Therapeutic Imagery and Dialogue, and acupuncture principles in severe cases.

Arthritis
Many types of arthritis respond well to a holistic and multi-disciplinary approach. We frequently employ acupuncture, nutrition and traditional manipulation as a general program. We have seen good response when a family member uses the CV-4 technique on the patient at home on a daily basis. The technique is easily taught to the caregiver. It requires about 15 minutes per day. The CV-4 technique improves the immune system and the removal of toxic wastes from the body. It is good for everyone.

Emotional Disorders
Some emotional disorders respond very well to CranioSacral Therapy. Depression is usually relieved with a specific set of

three craniosacral decompression techniques. One is applied to the low back and the other two are applied to specific areas of the head. Because of the specificity of treatment, this is best left in the hands of a therapist who has studied craniosacral work and has gained a significant degree of manual expertise.

Anxiety does not seem to have specific patterns. The still-point technique (CV-4) is very helpful in alleviating anxiety on a temporary basis, but the deep-seated causes must be resolved. The CV-4 technique is comparable to taking a pill. It gives temporary relief, but that doesn't solve the problem. SomatoEmotional Release will frequently get to the source of the anxiety.

Scoliosis

Scoliosis has many possible causes. Some of them are amenable to CranioSacral Therapy and some are not. Before one can predict the response, the cause must be discovered. The techniques used in CranioSacral Therapy and its related therapeutic approaches offer excellent means of discovery for these underlying causes of spinal curvature. Once the cause is known, the proper treatment approach can be considered.

Ear Problems

Chronic middle-ear infections respond exceedingly well to CranioSacral Therapy. Tinnitus (ringing in the ears) responds moderately well. It is more difficult to predict the results in tinnitus than it is in other ear problems.

Cerebral Ischemic Episodes (small strokes)

Cerebral Ischemic Episodes respond very well to weekly treatments of CranioSacral Therapy. We have seen great improvement in patients with memory loss, syncopy (fainting) and parethesias (strange sensations of body parts).

Visual Disturbances

Some visual and eye-motor (control) problems respond exceedingly well to CranioSacral Therapy and some do not; it depends on the cause. Nystagmus is a condition wherein the eyes just won't hold still. I have success in about 25 percent of these cases. Strabismus is the fancy name for crossed eyes. When the problem is due to nerve control of the eye muscle, we get better than 50 percent total improvement. Glaucoma is due to so many causes (remember the case of the lady who didn't want to see marital infidelity in mother, husband, etc.) that each has to be individually considered. We have had reasonably good results with improvement of visual acuity. Sometimes there is remarkable improvement and sometimes there is no effect at all. It depends on the reason for the problem.

25

Thank You CST-SER

This chapter, written in February, 1997, is an update to the original text of this book, which was written in 1990. My work with the craniosacral system began in the early 1970s. As my involvement with this system continued and deepened over the years, it kept my mind open and my thought processes innovative. In this chapter I have described some of the directions that I am traveling which I feel are at least partially, if not wholly, due to my involvement with the craniosacral system, its evaluation and treatment.

The major challenge is the adaptation required to work in so many areas concurrently. It is a wonderful lesson in keeping yourself open with a wide-spectrum focus. It requires the delegation of responsibility, which in turn requires the ability to trust. Through the processes that have entered my life since my first experiences with the craniosacral system, I have been shown that trust is the answer to so many of life's anxieties and worries. It is the thing that enables you to sleep at night when so many things are going on at once. Things that, without trust, might easily cause worry and insomnia.

Doing CranioSacral Therapy teaches trust. It teaches you to trust the craniosacral system, it teaches you to trust the inner wisdom of the patient or client, and it teaches you to trust yourself as the therapeutic facilitator. This work with

CST-SER also requires that you recognize those times when your ego is clouding your judgment. It requires that your ego be placed in proper perspective.

Join me as I describe some of the wonderful observations and events that have happened since the first chronicle of this journey was published.

Multiple-Hands/Multiple-Therapists Treatment

In our work we simply call this "multiple-hands" technique. What this means is that there are at least two therapists working at the same time on a single patient/client. More often, there are three or four therapists working as a team on one patient/client. There are times when I have worked with as many as 10 therapists on a single person. Most often, however, multiple hands means three or four therapists, which translates to six to eight therapeutic hands.

I was led into multiple-hands treatment through the use of my teaching methods. Since CranioSacral Therapy is a hands-on modality, it seemed to me that the best way to teach it would be to have the student's hands on the patient's/client's body as I worked, so that he or she (the student) could learn to feel and experience the bodily changes that were occurring in response to my applications of Cranio-Sacral Therapy techniques. The situation was reversed when it was time to evaluate the student's skill level. I might ask the student to carry out a given set of CranioSacral Therapy techniques while I monitored the patient's/client's bodily responses to the student's efforts.

Soon this interplay evolved to the level wherein I began to ask students to do certain techniques which would complement my own work with the patient at the same time. I began to realize that the work was much more effective and time-efficient when I asked the students to contribute rather than simply monitor.

Today (early 1997), multiple-hands work has evolved to the level wherein reasonably advanced CranioSacral Therapy practitioners work together on patients/clients in an almost telepathic way. Very few words may be spoken, but each member of the therapeutic team feels the same things, and the work of each therapist is almost always complementary to the total team effort. Most often, one therapist is the "team leader." This means that, if a treatment protocol question should arise, that team leader has the final say. Disagreements between therapists when they are working in the multiple-hands setting are extremely rare. Egos are most definitely subordinated when differences in approach or judgment might occur. Usually, a single word or two is enough to resolve any issues that may arise.

It has also become clear over the years that it is not at all necessary that the practitioners have even made each other's acquaintance before the treatment session begins. This is often the case in my own experience, because I conduct many tutorial-type seminars for groups of five or ten participants. These individuals may have come from distant parts of the country. Often, the small group may even be international. There may be a language barrier, but it seems not to matter very much. Usually, within a few minutes, therapists from the most divergent backgrounds and environments will be working as a single unit. It often reminds me of the days when I was working as a jazz piano player in order to get through school. Quite often, when we were to entertain in a club or play for a dance, three or four of us might meet each other for the first time as we were unpacking our instruments and getting ready to "tune up." We would play together for the next four to six hours. By the end of the night we usually felt like we had known each other for years. Usually, about halfway through the opening song, we were all pretty much on the same musical wavelength. If one of the group wasn't on that wavelength by the end of the first two or three songs, the chances were that he never would be, and his musical skills and/or musical tastes were not acceptable to the rest of the group. If this occurred, the rest of the night was "cover up" for the musician who just didn't fit in.

A similar bond develops in multiple-hands CranioSacral Therapy sessions. However, I believe that in CranioSacral Therapy groups the bond is stronger, it develops more quickly, there are fewer therapists who just don't "tune in" with the rest of the group, and the "telepathic" and "energetic" communications within the CranioSacral Therapy group are much stronger and more abundant than in the musical groups in which I participated.

Why do we do multiple-hands group treatment work? The main reason is that the patients/clients get better logarithmically faster and more effectively. I used to believe that I, working alone, could do everything for a patient/client that a group could accomplish doing multiple-hands. I don't believe that anymore. I have seen things happen with patients/clients that I am sure I could never accomplish working alone, no matter how long I worked at it.

There are a couple of reasons for this multiple-hands/multiple-therapist work being so much more effective. One is that the skills of each of the individual therapists seem to diffuse throughout the group. Each of us is more aware and more skilled working in group fashion as compared to working alone. It is as if a "pool of common knowledge" is created by the group of therapists, and each of us is then in possession of all the knowledge in the pool. Thus, the skill level does not simply increase in an additive fashion. It increases at least geometrically, if not logarithmically. The same seems true for the energy and intention of the group. At times, the effect of multiple-hands work seems almost miraculous. I am sure that if the same patient/client was treated by each individual therapist singularly, one right after the other, the therapeutic effect of the sequence of individual treatments would be much, much less than the effect of the multiple-hands session.

Clearly, multiple-hands treatment sessions cost more dollars immediately, but I truly believe that this type of work is cost-effective in the longer term. It is ideal for the difficult, chronic problems that have defied the usual methods of treatment.

CST-SER and PTSD CranioSacral Therapy — SomatoEmotional Release and Post-Traumatic Stress Disorder

Almost since the beginning of my relationship with Cranio-Sacral Therapy (CST) and SomatoEmotional Release (SER), I began seeing truly remarkable, positive results in patients/clients who were having nightmares, flashbacks, inability to concentrate, repetitive intrusive thoughts, blackouts and the like. Almost invariably during CST-SER treatment sessions, these people would release huge amounts of restrictive and foreign energies from their bodies.

Quite often they would re-experience severely traumatic incidents as they were re-experiencing the trauma. Sometimes they recalled the trauma later on. The recall could occur in a dream that night, or it could appear in total or in a number of smaller pieces a day, a week, a month or even a year later. Most often the recall would come into their conscious awareness either during the session or within a day or so. It was quite common for these memories to come forward with only moderate emotional impact. It seemed as though the release of the body energy took a significant amount of the power out of the traumatic memory.

One might theorize that the memory of the traumatic incident was totally suppressed by a part of the mind whose purpose it was to spare the patient/client the unbearable recall of the incident. However, the cost of suppression was high and the suppression was not totally effective, as evidenced by the nightmares, etc.

After these sessions of energy release and the recall into consciousness of the traumatic incidents, the symptoms abated and the improvement in the quality of life and ability to perform were quite remarkable. In my own experience, patient after patient came to me. They went through the CST-SER process and were relieved of the burdens that they were carrying. It should be emphasized here that I was not directing and not suggesting that traumatic experiences might be the cause of the problem to any of these patients. The releases and recalls all came forward from within the patients, without urging from me. When images began to come forward I did verbally encourage the process by simply saying such things as "go on," "keep going," "I'm with you," and the like. I wanted to let them know that they were not alone and that they were doing well.

After it was clear to me that this CST-SER process was quite effective, I began to teach it to more advanced CST students. Reports of successful treatment of rape victims, satanic cult victims, child abuse victims, survivors of catastrophic phenomena, etc., kept rolling in. During this same time the concept of Post-Traumatic Stress Disorder (PTSD) was being formalized and accepted as a bona fide psychoemotional or brain function disorder. It seemed that we were treating these PTSD patients with a significant degree of success.

A little digging into statistics revealed that over 2.5 million American soldiers had been deployed in the Vietnam conflict. Of this group, about 500,000 were involved in active combat. At the time that we did our digging, the guesses were that perhaps 250,000 of these soldiers were still experiencing the symptoms of PTSD. These symptoms included frequent and repetitive nightmares, repetitive flashbacks triggered by a wide variety of stimuli, inability to feel emotions, inability to form emotional attachments, suspicion and paranoia, hostility (sometimes uncontrollable), hyperarousal which often manifested as a perpetual state of readiness to engage in "defensive" acts of violence, depression, sexual dysfunction, social alienation, substance abuse and addictions, and with all of this, of course, there is a very high rate of spousal abuse and divorce. More recent surveys by the Veterans Administration, as of 1996, reflect that the VA hospitals and clinics presently have about 26,000 patients in active therapy. These patients had well over 300,000 outpatient visits. The results have been poor in terms of relief of symptoms and/or rehabilitation, or re-entry into society.

From the aforementioned description, you can see the picture and the need. I decided that we should put the CST-SER treatment process to the test. We had connection with one Vietnam veteran who was suffering severely from his PTSD problem. He, in turn, convinced five other PTSD sufferers to participate. Four of them had been in VA treatment programs for several years. The other participant had not accepted VA treatment by choice, but she suffered significantly.

I set up a two-week intensive treatment program which took place in March, 1993. We used 18 therapists for the six patients. We began work every day at 10 a.m. and provided CST-SER treatment for each veteran for as long as it seemed appropriate. Usually the end of the day was between 5 and 6 p.m. We had all six of the veterans housed at a small ocean-front motel along with about six of the therapists who had come some distance to participate.

I won't go into the details of the treatment process here because that could be another book. Suffice it to say that all six did extremely well. We videotaped interviews by a neutral psychiatrist at the beginning and the end of the two-week program individually, for each of the veterans. We had good follow-up for a year on all six of them. And we are still in touch with three of them on a current basis, over three years later. Four of the veterans are now gainfully employed and feeling good. One was killed in an automobile accident as he was returning from attending a CranioSacral Therapy seminar. He had decided to train to become a CST practitioner and work with other PTSD veterans. He would have been fabulous at this job. The other veteran still lapses into an occasional alcoholic spree. But he has not used any other drugs, nor has he attempted suicide since the program. Prior to our treatment program he had three serious suicide attempts on his record and was using cocaine fairly regularly, with some heroine usage interspersed.

CST-SER as a treatment modality for one of the worst kinds of PTSD had passed the preliminary tests with flying colors. At present, we are trying hard to find sponsorship for more treatment programs, and as soon as possible, a training program for interested therapists. The two weeks of treatment is very labor intensive. The multiple-hands work with the CST-SER approach is essential. All of this makes the whole thing look very expensive. On the other hand, I wonder what it had cost for the previous, rather ineffective treatments that the four totally rehabilitated veterans had undergone prior to their participation in our program. I know it hasn't cost much, if anything, since that time. We do need support to implement and continue this program. Help!!!

The Float Tank

It was sometime in the summer of 1984 when a friend invited me over to have a session in an isolation tank that he had installed in the living room of his ocean-view, eighth floor condominium. I had read about isolation tanks in some of John Lilly, M.D.'s, writings some years earlier. I accepted the invitation and, after having been suspended upside down by my feet in his inversion-boot apparatus for 20 minutes, I took a thorough shower to eliminate skin oil and perspiration. I was then put into a tank which resembled a rather spacious coffin, lid and all. I have never forgotten the strange sensation as I met the buoyancy of the water with my foot when I stepped over the side and into the tank. I literally had to push my foot down to the bottom of the tank. The water in the tank was about 18 inches deep. It was extremely buoyant because it was a solution of Epsom salt (magnesium sulfate) which was concentrated to about 50 percent.

My friend instructed me to simply lie on top of the water on my back and relax, but make sure I didn't get the water in my eyes because it would burn. I also discovered that a drop or two of the Epsom salt water in your mouth did not taste very good. It was amazing. I laid on the water. Immediately, I felt the freedom in my body that resulted from the virtual neutralization of the forces of gravity, and the freedom from the friction to which your skin is subjected when you try to slide into a different position as you are lying down on a bed, a couch, a floor, etc. I could feel muscles begin to relax almost immediately. Many of these are muscles that, unbeknownst to us on a conscious level, are constantly working to balance the forces of gravity as we stand, sit, lie, walk, rollerblade, dance, etc.

Then my friend closed the lid of the tank. The darkness was uninterrupted. There was no sound except for the ones I might have made by splashing the water a bit, or with my own voice. I also became quite aware of some of the sounds of peristalsis in my gastrointestinal tract as I settled into this "gravity-free" environment. I listened to myself breath and, a little later, I listened to my heart beating.

This awareness of my "self" and my body parts and functions ultimately led me into an "altered state" of profound relaxation. Time was no longer in my equation as I began simply to exist. At some point my body began to make fish-like movements, as though my pelvis and legs were the lower part of a fish moving its tail from side to side. This movement was nice and easy. The neurophysiologist in me related these movements to an expression of what we call "reciprocal innervation." The principle here is that, when your trunk is bent to the side in one direction past a certain threshold, the muscles on the other side of the trunk contract. In doing so, the nerve impulses are diverted from the side to which you are bent, and those muscles relax. Your trunk now bends in the opposite direction until that side-bending threshold is passed. The nerve impulses are then diverted again to the opposite side, causing muscle contraction and side bending in that direction.

The side-to-side activity went on and on in a very lazy and relaxed way. Each bend seemed to achieve further relaxation of my trunk muscles.

Several times my vertebrae gave out popping sounds, much as you hear during a spinal manipulation. It was a marvelous experience. All too soon, my friend opened the lid and I was out of the tank and back in the world of gravitational pulls and invasive sights and sounds. I had been in the isolation tank for an hour and 20 minutes. My body felt loose and flexible. However, as I walked, showered, dressed, etc., I could feel some of the old tension patterns making their presence known again as the struggle with gravity was resumed.

What has this to do with CranioSacral Therapy? First of all, very deep CranioSacral Therapy often creates similar sensations of relaxation in your body. It also, quite frequently, puts the patient/client into a rather altered state of consciousness that is very relaxing and, I believe, a time to heal. The big question came into my mind long ago, but it wasn't until about 1990 that I had the time and resources to seriously consider it: What happens when you combine CranioSacral Therapy with a flotation tank experience?

After a bit of shopping, I found a company that would build a tank to my specifications. I wanted a working area inside of the tank that would accommodate a patient/client lying on the water, and room for up to six therapists working with this patient/client. We built a tank that was six-feet wide and 10-feet long. It accommodated a water level up to 30 inches. It was so constructed that it could be soundproof and light proof, as we desired. The Epsom salt solution was maintained at about 50 percent concentration. The water was held at a constant temperature of 96 degrees Fahrenheit. The water was filtered and treated with ozone daily.

We worked with a few patients who had suffered strokes, head injuries and spinal cord injuries. All were paralyzed to some degree. It is my feeling that paralyzed people suffering from either brain or spinal cord problems probably also receive some contribution to their paralytic condition from the muscles that have been either spastic, injured, hypertonic and/or unused. Our intent was to work with the craniosacral system while being in the flotation tank. This allowed us to work with the muscles, joints, ligaments, fascias, etc., in a virtually gravity-free and friction-free environment. Our results were very encouraging. It seems true that some of the paralytic condition is self-perpetuated by the peripheral musculoskeletal system, even though the brain and spinal cord may be improving. We were able to find very subtle "trigger" areas with the patient/client floating in the tank that we would never have found while under the influence of gravity. When we found these areas and released the spasticity in them, we usually saw significant improvement in function and patient comfort.

We also treated patients/clients with post-operative adhesions in the abdomen, in the chest after coronary bypass surgeries, and in the legs and groin where veins were taken surgically in order to be used as materials for the bypass surgeries. In these adhesion cases we were able to pinpoint the locations of the adhesions and release them using the buoyancy of the water as a therapeutic tool. For intra-abdominal adhesions, we could quite often simply hold the patient's/client's pelvis forcibly at the floor of the tank. The buoyancy of the water solution seems to cause the internal organs to try to float towards the top of the water even though they are inside of the body. We then used this floating tendency as a kind of internally applied traction. By positioning the body correctly, we saw clinical results that would indicate that the adhesions had been released.

As we progressed in our exploration we found that we used the isolation from sound and light less and less and, finally, not at all. The CranioSacral Therapy was producing a relaxed state that was more effective than that which was produced by isolation from sound and light. Release from the isolation aspect allowed the therapists to be better able to work effectively.

Our tank has recently suffered some deterioration problems, so we are without it at present. We miss it very much, and a new tank is on the drawing board. It will be a little larger because we often use five or six therapists with one patient/client in order to obtain maximum results. We have found that the ability to offer more freedom of movement is important. Patients/clients who have been spastically paralyzed for a significant period of time benefit from a sort of "free-unwinding" process during the treatment. We will not bother with the isolation aspect of the flotation tank. What really helps is a good multiple-hands team in warm Epsom salt water that won't let gravity be a consideration in the equation. I also strongly suspect that the abundance of magnesium ions in the solution has a positive effect.

As in multiple-hands work, the cost of using the flotation tank is higher but the results are better and quicker. Therefore, the patient/client has fewer healthcare costs later on.

Getting Grounded

Grounding has many meanings. In the bodywork community, grounding usually means taking a moment to clear your mind of extraneous and intrusive thoughts, getting energies centered and in synchrony. It means focusing upon what you are about to do with the patient/client that is before you.

Here I use "body" in reference to the human body, not the automobile body. In physics and electricity, grounding means something different, but it is perhaps somewhat analogous. It means the use of a conductor such as a wire to carry an electrical charge into the earth. This is the principle of lightening rods, and so on. Little did I ever guess that I would be using both of these types of groundings on certain patients. I always take a few seconds to do the first type of grounding as I enter the room for a treatment session. I did not suspect that I would ever be grounding some of these patients in the electrophysics sense of the word.

168

Here is the story: About five years ago a circuit court judge came to see me. He was suffering from intractable headaches. I did whole-body evaluation, time after time, and always came up with excess energy in the total spinal cord and/or spinal vertebrae. I could not localize it any better than that. And it did not feel like a typical kind of restriction to motion. It felt all disorganized and overactive. The only time I had felt any energy of this quality before was in a young man who had been electrocuted by a 220-volt wire. He was in coma for a few days and hospitalized for a week or so. I saw him during my research work at Michigan State University. His energy was also disorganized and hyperactive. It was like that all through his body. I could not localize the problem nearly as well as I did with the judge.

As I recall, I had only two more electrocution patients between that first young man and the judge. I did fairly well, just trying to drain off their excess energy through my own body. In both cases the symptomatic improvement, mostly arthritic-type pain, was about 50 to 75 percent. But I knew intuitively that this was a very inefficient treatment method. Also, it exhausted me, and I had a lot of aches and pains for a few hours subsequent to each treatment.

The judge had not been electrocuted and the energy was essentially in a line from his tailbone to the top of his head. In terms of headache relief, we were getting nowhere. Then he said the magic words, "It feels like an electric shock, a bolt of lightening that goes from my tail to my head when the headache hits me. And I never know when it is going to happen."

I believe in following my intuition, and something told me to ground him in the electrophysics sense. He had a rather severe headache at that time. I connected his big toe to the drain pipe under the sink by a copper wire. Within minutes his headache began to subside. Concurrently, the disorganized and hyperactive energy that I had been feeling subsided. His craniosacral system, which had been hard to evaluate, seemed to normalize. The relief only lasted about 36 hours, then the headaches resumed. I used the wire grounding again and it worked.

The judge lived a long distance away. I had no idea what caused his initial problem, but we did find out that he could get control of the situation by literally grounding himself. He bought a four-foot length of half-inch copper pipe and used it as a walking stick on the ground, not on the sidewalk. I heard from him about six months later and he was still doing well.

Since the judge, I have treated two headache patients successfully by grounding them. Now comes the good part. There is a medical condition called "reflex sympathetic dystrophy." It is synonymous with severe, almost unbearable pain. There is no effective treatment for it. We had a lady about 40 years old come to us from a distance with this type of unrelenting pain. She was seen by one of my colleagues, Dr. Lisa Squier, who I have since married.

Lisa asked if I would consult with her on this patient because the patient could not stand to be touched. In our approach, if we can't touch the patient our most used modality is gone. I saw the patient and evaluated her without touching her, just sensing her bodily energy field. Her energy was very hot, very powerful, and if I brought my hand within three or four inches of her body she would scream with pain. Wearing clothes gave her great pain. (In France, I had seen a patient with similar pain subsequent to a stroke in the thalamus.) In this lady's case, the onset occurred right after a surgical procedure on her left arm, which had been injured in an automobile accident. Over a period of weeks after the surgery, her pain had progressed to the level we saw at the time of her visit to us.

I thought of grounding her with the wire, so I did. Within 10 minutes we could touch her without hearing a scream. I then did acupuncture for total body pain, and we moved down another notch in terms of her discomfort. To make a long story short, by the use of copper-wire grounding and acupuncture, we were able to determine that the problem was an abnormally high nerve impulse input from the arm into a major sympathetic nervous system ganglion at the junction of the neck and the upper back on the left side. This is called the stellate ganglion. From there, the whole pain sensory system was hyperactivated.

She went home in reasonably good condition after two weeks of daily treatment. Her husband grounded her to a sink drain on a 30-foot wire so she could get around the house. She returned for more treatment in about six weeks and has made two more visits to us since that time. Each visit is two weeks. She is here as I write this description. She has residual pain at the surgical site in her left arm, in her left hand and in her shoulder. Otherwise, she is happy and pain-free. We want to get the left arm completely free of pain and mobile so that the danger of recurrence of whole-body reflex sympathetic dystrophy becomes nonexistent. She has not used the grounding wire since her second series of treatments with us. Our main focus now is to restore freedom of motion to her bodily tissues.

Since this patient, we have had two more reflex sympathetic dystrophy patients who responded to grounding, and some others that did not require it. It makes some sense, if you consider that the nervous system makes electrical potential. If it makes too much and does not have a means of dealing with the excess, some of it will stimulate pain receptors. We simply drain the excess electrical potential by grounding, and then search for and correct the cause of the excess production.

When Divers Get Dizzy

The lore amongst the world-class divers has it that, once a diver gets dizzy, it is time to start looking for another career. When you consider the tremendous number of significant pressure changes their bodies are subjected to during their training and the actual competitions, it does seem reasonable that their balance mechanisms might get confused. After all, the pressure changes go into the ear, and it is in the inner ear chamber that the very delicate equilibrium system is located.

Mary Ellen Clark won the bronze medal for the 10-meter platform dive in the summer Olympic games in Atlanta, Georgia. When I first saw her in mid-September, 1995, at The Upledger Institute, Inc., HealthPlex Clinical Services, she had about given up on making the next Olympic games as an athlete. She had been unable to train for about a year prior because she had developed a severe case of vertigo. It was so bad that at times, before she stopped diving, she was confused upon entering the water. She was so confused that sometimes she swam to the bottom of the pool instead of swimming to the top. In her words, she had "been everywhere and done everything to get better. Nothing helped." There seemed to be no solution to her problem. It seemed that every time she dove it got worse. So she and her coach decided she would stop diving.

During our first session, Mary Ellen told the long story of her experiences with a wide variety of healthcare approaches. But I let it go in one ear and out the other. When you want to find the cause of a problem, you start fresh. You cannot allow yourself to be influenced by other people's/doctor's opinions. If they had found the true answer, the chances are that this patient before you would have no need to see you.

I completed my whole-body evaluation using just my hands to evaluate the mobility of the tissues throughout her body. I was looking for areas of restriction, and in my search I disregarded her symptoms. I found several significant Energy Cysts within her torso that would most likely have resulted from traumatic blows to her body. I released these Energy Cysts quite easily. She confirmed that in her practice sessions she frequently hit the water on her back, her belly, her side, etc., while learning a new dive. Her collisions with the water were at speeds of about 35 miles per hour. If you have ever done a belly flop from just a few feet above water level you may recall how hard the water is when you strike it with a relatively flat part of your body. Mary Ellen said that during her training she would often do 50 dives per day. So she hit the water 50 times each day at 35 miles per hour, and about 10 percent of the time she hit the water inappropriately. Also, she went down into the water about 15 to 16 feet with each dive. That is quite a pressure change on the whole body, especially the head with its ear openings. I suppose this is why most of the medical attention had been focused on her ears as an entry to her equilibrium apparatus.

During that first session we cleared most of the torso Energy Cysts. At the next session my whole-body evaluation pointed to her left knee. She confirmed that she had seriously "wrenched" her knee during a trampoline accident while practicing the various body twists, etc., that were part of a new dive she was learning. She had paid little attention to the knee injury. I suspect she could do this because she was so accomplished at denying the presence of pain. As things developed, it became clear that the knee injury had caused her to compensate with her pelvis and low back. The pelvis was pulled up on the left side. Her spine twisted to compensate, which caused her head to be improperly positioned on her neck. As we focused on the correction of these problems and their sequelae, which were found mostly in the right occiput and temporal bone, she began to improve. I saw her weekly, and by the end of October she was able to resume some of her physical conditioning work but not her high platform diving, as yet.

At the beginning of each session I did whole-body evaluation so that we could work that day on the areas suggested by her bodily restrictions and energy patterns. Soon it became apparent that her symptoms could be subdivided into two subcategories, namely vertigo and light-headedness. I could reproduce her vertigo by using very light manual pressure in a specific direction on her right temporal bone. I could cause the right temporal bone to make the same movement and cause the dizziness by moving her sacrum a certain way. The light-headedness was reproducible by side-bending her head to the right on the top cervical vertebrae. I could also cause this symptom to occur when I moved her pelvis further into the compensatory pattern related to the left knee problem, and/or when I rotated her lumbar spine in a given manner. Now that the situation had revealed itself, we both felt very encouraged. It was a rather straightforward use of CST, Energy Cyst Release, manipulation of the knee, spinal manipulation, pelvic rebalancing and myofascial release that has totally corrected the problem. By the end of December, 1995, she was able to resume a full training schedule, and as you saw if you watched the Olympic games, she did a beautiful job and won the bronze medal.

Both Mary Ellen and I know that her problem would not have been resolved had we not done whole-body evaluation at the beginning of each session and followed the leads obtained.

Whole-body evaluation requires the practitioner to set aside anything previously known about the patient/client during this evaluation. The clues and cues that we seek during whole-body evaluation are extremely subtle. Previous biases and experiences with a patient/client can cause evaluators to imagine that they feel what they expect to find, based on these previous experiences. In my experience, each session is a new experience and I like to pretend that each is a first-time patient. That way we keep finding new and pertinent things.

Remember, all living things are in a state of dynamic change. Our biggest errors in healthcare are sometimes based upon previous situations and the assumption that what was true of a person yesterday is true today. Others are based upon the acceptance of previous findings by others, and/or by the acceptance of the "obvious," which was true in Mary Ellen's case.

It's Music to His Back

Crafton accepted the position as conductor of a local Pops Orchestra in early 1996. He is a young man of 38 years. He endures rather severe pain in his back, both in the upper and lower regions, almost every day of his life. It has been going on for a long time. Prior to coming to Florida he conducted a Cincinnati orchestra. He was referred to me by his physical therapist in Cincinnati, who had been working with him for a couple of years. Crafton had received temporary relief in Cincinnati, but no true permanent improvement.

I first saw Crafton in May of 1996. We had only this one session. He called and said he felt great for a couple of weeks but within a month the pain had returned in full force. Our schedules did not match up very well. I have a very full schedule, he traveled a lot, etc. I really wasn't sure that I had done him any good because he didn't come back. Then in December he called and offered me tickets to an evening with the Pops Orchestra, so Lisa and I went. He invited us backstage to visit with him during the first intermission. During the visit he confessed that time was one problem, travel was another, money was a third factor, but he really did want to get back to see me because he did feel quite good for awhile.

As I listened to this very kind and artistic person tell his story, an idea came into my head. It had to do with some experimenting I had done with another doctor over in Amsterdam where I was teaching. I had long been thinking about the potential resonance of tissues to certain sound waves and their frequencies. My intuition said that a cello had the proper quality and range to investigate whether certain notes might cause resonant tissue reactions in human bodies. My Dutch doctor friend, Jan van Dixhoorn, was a cardiologist who also played classical cello. We tried our experiment on several friends and volunteers. Sure enough, as Jan played the scales chromatically on the cello, I could feel changes in tissue tensions and energy patterns in the subject's body, as well as feel the effects of certain notes on the amplitude and quality of the rhythmical activity of the craniosacral system. When I returned home there was lots of other work to do and no competent cellist available, so the idea was set on the back burner.

As I listened to Crafton talking, I realized that this might be something he could try for his back pain. I asked whether he could recruit one of his cellists to come to my home with him, where we could explore the possibility that certain notes could be used to provide him relief from back pain.

It is only about two weeks ago as I write the account of these events that Crafton came to our home with a wonderful cellist named Liz. The sounds that she produced from her instrument were absolutely beautiful and pure. As she ascended and descended the scales, I monitored the tissues of

Crafton's back with my hands and also did an "arcing" procedure for confirmation. The arcing is done from a distance on the body, usually the feet. With practice, the evaluator is able to detect the vibrational energy outputs throughout the body and tell which areas are out of synchrony. When these tissues realign energetically, the arcing pattern disappears.

To make a rather long story short, both direct palpation and arcing confirmed the positive effects upon muscle relaxation when both open G and B were played. The open G (no finger on the G string) was the most effective in both the upper and lower back problems. The B was effective only in the upper back. As Liz continued to play the note, Crafton could feel the muscle tissues relaxing and the pain going away. So, our idea was to have one of the cellists play his "therapeutic" notes for him on a daily basis to see whether or not we might achieve a more acceptable repatterning of his back muscle tensions. This approach is aimed at relief and possible reprogramming.

Now, another very interesting observation. We found that concert A caused his back muscles to tighten up, and his pain to begin and continually increase as long as Liz played the A. You may have guessed it by now: A is the note played by the whole orchestra when they tune up. We'll see how it all works out, but I suspect that Crafton may have his orchestra tune to a different note. This really opens some doors for investigation, doesn't it?

Working With Dolphins

It was in 1954 when I had my first rather intimate interaction with dolphins. To be honest, I'm not sure whether they were dolphins or porpoises. But they are very close kin to each other, so I'm not sure that it matters much. One of the trainers I met agreed to call them dolpoises or porphins. For our purposes (porpoises) we'll refer to them as dolphins.

In any case, from mid-1954 until September, 1956, I had the pleasure of serving as the "medic" aboard a U.S. Coast Guard air-sea rescue cutter, which was home-based in Panama City, Florida. We patrolled the Gulf of Mexico 10 out of every 30 days, and were on call for rescue work at either 30-minute or two-hour standby throughout the 20 days in port. As it turned out, we were out in the Gulf at least half of the time. We were constantly accompanied by large numbers of dolphins. Often they would rub their backs on the hull of our ship as we were cruising, usually between 10 and 15 miles per hour. They played and made spiral patterns with each other most of the time.

On reasonably calm days when we were perhaps 50 or 100 miles from shore, at about 4:00 p.m. the "skipper" would often announce over the loud speaker that it was "swim call." We were a small ship, 125 feet in length, and the sides of the deck were only about three or four feet above water level, so it wasn't any big deal to dive or jump over the side when the announcement was made. I grew up in Detroit. I swam in the Detroit River and Lake St. Clair, as well as several smaller lakes and gravel pits near Detroit. I knew nothing of salt water except what I had read and seen in movies.

The first time I heard this announcement I noted that a gunner's mate was manning our 20 millimeter. (To us, this was a "cannon" because the largest gun we had was 40 millimeters, and this was considered our "big cannon." The Coast Guard, in those days, was not equipped for combat.) I asked why he was up there. The reply was "to protect the swimmers against any sharks that might come around." I didn't think this was anything more than a token defense. Nonetheless, probably half of our 40-man crew jumped into the water. (The ship was either anchored or drifting during swim calls.) I noted that immediately upon their entry into the water, they were surrounded by dolphins.

I had heard somewhere that sharks were afraid of dolphins, and being a "macho" Detroiter with a reputation for toughness to uphold, I too jumped in the water. It was a very strange thing that then happened. I was almost immediately "escorted" by two dolphins. I was quite fearful when I went in the Gulf, but there was a pride issue involved, so I did it. It was as though the dolphins sensed my fear and sympathized with me. With a dolphin on my left and a dolphin on my right I felt my fear immediately disappear. Those wonderful dolphins were immediately there for all of us when we jumped into the water. It was as though they heard the swim-call announcement and decided to make sure that we were safe.

Quite often we were called upon to board fishing vessels out in the middle of the Gulf. We usually did this by small boat, using oars. There were always dolphins with us when we made these rowing expeditions. During the two years I was aboard the Coast Guard Cutter Cartigan, I would guess that I did swim call far out in the Gulf of Mexico at least 75 to 100 times, and probably participated in row-boat ventures between our ship and other vessels, in fairly rough waters, about 50 times. I cannot recall a time when we did not have dolphin escorts. I simply felt safe with them around.

In 1964 I opened my private practice of osteopathic medicine and surgery on Clearwater Beach on the west coast of Florida. I was there over 11 years, about four of which were spent in houses directly on the Gulf beach. The rest of the time we lived perhaps five to 10 minutes from the beach. Being in the Gulf water, both swimming and sailing a small boat, was a large part of my recreation. I had many, many friendly encounters with dolphins during those years. I learned to accept their friendship and an almost palpable love. I trusted them implicitly.

Many times they could have overwhelmed me, either while I was swimming or sailing. But although untrained, they were always playful but very careful. They seemed to know how fragile I was in comparison to them. They also understood that water was not my primary environment, and respected my needs as a landlubber, and the restrictions that water imposed upon me. I began to know, intuitively, that within the soul of each dolphin I met was a very wise and powerful ability to "heal" others and to understand our needs and pains. I also understood that the dolphins care a great deal about us humans, although we as a species have done precious little to deserve this love and consideration.

The seeds were planted. I began to hope that at some point in my life I would have the opportunity to develop a working relationship with one or more dolphins in the practice of healthcare. I had no idea how or when this might occur, but I had the idea planted deep in my brain somewhere. Then came my move to Michigan State University and the dolphin idea was set aside. Fortunately, the delay was temporary, and perhaps served a purpose by allowing me the time to learn and grow to a level wherein I was more ready to work with these marvelous beings.

Before I get into our present work with dolphins, I think it might help you to appreciate the "wisdom" of dolphins by relating an experience described to me over dinner by Timothy Wyllie, who has had significant time and experience with dolphins. Timothy wrote about some of his experiences and ideas in a book entitled The Deta Factor. It seems that Timothy was staying on the Gulf beach near Sarasota, Florida, for a few months while doing some writing.

He became fascinated with dolphins and began to interact with them as he swam in the Gulf every evening, just before sundown. He got the idea that, were he to get into trouble while swimming, the dolphins would come to his rescue. He became so taken with the idea that he decided to test it. He swam out into the Gulf and pretended to founder. A few dolphins circled him, but did not help him. He understood that they knew he was pretending.

The next night he did something that could be called many things, among them stupid, foolhardy, courageous, determined, obsessive, trusting, etc. He swam out into the Gulf until he could no longer swim any further. He was truly foundering this time. The dolphins knew it. Three of them came to his rescue and took him back to shallow water. One dolphin was either beneath or behind him — the dolphin kept changing position. Two dolphins gave their dorsal fins to his hands, one on each side, and "towed" him in to water about three feet deep, where all three took their leave after being sure that he could stand and wade in towards shore.

I shall never forget this story. It served to confirm my own intuitive feelings about what could happen if we were to work side by side in the water with them.

In September, 1996, after almost a year of negotiation, we opened a program at the Dolphin Research Center in Grassy Key, Florida, wherein we treated patients in the water along with dolphins. We were in water about three to four feet deep so that the therapists could stand while working. The patients were floating on top of the water assisted by flotation devices that offered minimal obstruction to access of the patients' bodies, either by the dolphins or by the therapists. The patients were mostly significantly disabled persons. The disabilities were either subsequent to disease or injury. One therapist was placed at each patient's head, one at the feet and a third at the pelvis. They were all highly skilled in CranioSacral Therapy (CST) and SomatoEmotional Release (SER).

The treatment sessions were conducted as typical CST-SER multiple-hands sessions and the dolphins were free to enter and participate as they chose. We deliberately left one side of each patient open for dolphin approach. Sometimes they used this opening and sometimes not. We always sent thoughts out that invited the dolphin to enter and participate as he or she saw fit. I would allow no directing of dolphin behavior related to the actual treatment. At times the trainers gave directions, but only related to which patient a given dolphin should work with. Very soon these directions were minimized, and frequently dolphins were allowed to make their own choices. Our therapists silently encouraged this freedom of choice. I also insisted that each therapist hold the attitude that the dolphin was at least equal to them in knowledge and skill, and probably superior. This attitude on our part was soon perceived by the dolphins, and they became very creative in their treatment processes.

Typically, the dolphins would circle the patient-therapist group in the water. After a few circlings were made, one of the dolphins would approach, very gently, and either touch a therapist or the patient with his or her nose (rostrum). All of us would feel very powerful energy from the dolphin. This might occur five or 10 times, then the dolphin would be through. This process might be followed by a treatment of the patient upon the dock, and then another session in the water with the dolphins.

The therapeutic results were often quite remarkable. A young lady with a crooked pelvis and a short right leg was treated. I was on the pelvis and I had my two assistant therapists, one on the patient's head and one on her feet. My goal for this session was to gain some loosening of the injured pelvis and some correction of its central control system in the brain. The dolphin joined us and never touched the patient. She put her rostrum on the backs of the two assistant therapists (one at a time, of course), between the shoulder blades, about half a dozen times on each. The duration of the dolphin's contact was perhaps a minute or less each time. During each of these dolphin contact times, we all felt significant but pleasant vibrations throughout the patient's body. Also, each time the dolphin contacted one of the assistant therapists, I felt the patient's pelvis release and soften. Upon coming out of the water we re-measured the leg length difference. Before the dolphin session the right leg was about three inches longer than the left. After the session the difference in leg length was only about one inch. The patient felt a lot of pain-relief during and after the dolphin session. Another young girl used her paralyzed right arm to help herself climb the ladder out of the lagoon after her session.

From what I have seen and participated in I want very much to continue this exploratory work with dolphins. At this time we are wide open to carrying on this work at multiple locations concurrently. If you have an interest in sponsorship, please contact me via fax or mail. Include a brief description of what might be available.

As an added bonus in this dolphin project, all of our CST practitioners who have participated in the water with the dolphins (and there have been 23 therapists who have participated) have stated that their own skill levels were enhanced in some nonconscious way by their association with the dolphins in a therapeutic setting in the water. I know my own level of treatment skill has definitely improved. I would go on the record as saying that the dolphins, when allowed and encouraged to make their own creative choices, are not only powerful therapeutic facilitators, they are fantastically effective teachers.

CranioSacral Therapy, Obstetrics and Pediatrics

When I left my private practice on Clearwater Beach, Florida, to join the faculty at Michigan State University, one of the first surprises came from the Genessee County Director of Special Education. He told me that he estimated that about one in twenty (five percent) of the children in Michigan's public school system suffered from some sort of brain dysfunction. Whether or not his estimate is totally accurate, it calls your attention to the possibility that there may be a lot of brain-dysfunctioning children in the Michigan public school system. If he was close to correct, and if Michigan is a relatively typical state, imagine how many children may be brain dysfunctional, in one way or another, in the whole country. I have listed many of the types of brain dysfunction previously in this book.

During the first year or two of my research on the craniosacral system and its level of function in children, I became convinced that about half of these children could be significantly helped by CranioSacral Therapy. I also became convinced that a very significant percentage (probably about 50 percent) of these CST candidates could have had effective correction of their craniosacral system problems accomplished within the first week after their deliveries, and thus avoided the problems imposed by brain dysfunction as they matured.

It became clear to me that several of the brain-dysfunction problems were secondary to the difficulties encountered by the fetus in the mother's uterus and/or during the delivery process, and/or very shortly thereafter. I began campaigning in the late '70s for the use of craniosacral evaluation and treatment, either in the delivery room or in the newborn nursery in the case of hospital deliveries, and, of course, by midwives or other healthcare professionals in the case of home deliveries.

If CranioSacral Therapy (CST) is used for the mother during the pregnancy, much of the physiological stress can be eased. Also, the muscular, connective tissue and bony adaptations can be facilitated. Through the use of CST combined with SomatoEmotional Release (SER), many of the emotional issues that may be related to the pregnancy can be resolved. My feeling is that the emotions of the mother are "absorbed" by the fetus in the uterus. We have treated many children and adults who would seem to have an unwarranted emotional problem that ultimately resolved when the realization occurred that the emotion was the mother's and had been taken on by the fetus in the womb. Often, these emotional problems involve guilt that the mother felt, perhaps about the pregnancy, or anger at the father who did not want the child, and so on. By the time of the birth the mother may have resolved the guilt or anger which may have been caused by temporary conditions or misunderstandings. However, during the time when the emotional episode was active, the fetus absorbed and kept the emotion. These emotions can be released from both the mother and fetus before the delivery, or from the mother and child very soon after delivery. In so doing, many years of guilt, anger, etc., might be avoided.

In the past two or three years, there have been several inquiries from hospital personnel and, more recently, from hospital administrators regarding the use of CST and SER in the labor rooms, the obstetrical delivery suites and in the newborn nurseries. If this can be implemented, I am sure that we will see a reduction in colic, strabismus, cerebral palsy, seizure problems, respiratory problems, sensory and motor defects, as well as a variety of other brain dysfunctions in infants. As the generation of CST-treated children reach the grade schools, I am also sure that we will see a reduction in the percentage of learning-disabled and speech-impaired children.

Based on the possible introduction of CST and SER into conventional obstetrics and pediatrics, we have begun specialized training programs for CST-SER practitioners in the treatment of pregnant women and infants. I have the feeling that once the first hospital makes it official, there are many others that will follow suit in the use of these modalities in the obstetrical and pediatric departments. Many are now using them unofficially. It is time to come out of the closet. It reminds me of the days when I played with dance bands to support my schooling. Very often the dance floor remained unused through the first several songs that we played. Suddenly, when only one couple came out on the dance floor, within seconds the dance floor was full.

At this point I would like to share two letters that typify the kind of experiences expectant mothers have had with CST and SER surrounding their pregnancies and/or relating to residual effects of incomplete pregnancies. The first is from Pam Markert, a physical therapist and CranioSacral Therapy practitioner. Pam encouraged me to use her name and to print the letter as she wrote it. The second letter I have edited and kept the name of the author anonymous in order to protect her privacy. Both letters are self-explanatory.

Dear Dr. Upledger:

I am writing to thank you for all your pioneering work with CranioSacral Therapy. It has made a profound difference in my life, both personally and professionally. I would like to share my personal experience with you.

Back in the early '90s my husband and I wanted to start a family. Although I had undergone surgery when I was 12 years old for removal of a paraovarian cyst and one fallopian tube, my doctor did not feel I would have trouble conceiving. After a couple of years of trying and some medical testing that was negative, I decided to try cranial work. During a pelvic diaphragm release, a restriction along the incisional area was discovered and released. Following that treatment my menstrual cramps were minimal and I no longer needed prescription medication for the pain. We conceived the following month without any further intervention of any kind.

During my pregnancy I was plagued by "morning" sickness that lasted 24 hours a day. Fortunately for me I was attending a craniosacral course at the time and received a couple of treatments. My morning sickness disappeared immediately. Following the course it returned somewhat, unfortunately, but I suspect, had I been able to have a bit more work done, it may have completely abated and not returned. It still amazes me how good I felt after the treatment, when prior to that I could have felt so awful. I am grateful that the morning sickness never returned to the level it had been prior to the treatment.

As my pregnancy advanced I began to develop a constant right-sided headache, as well as right lumbosacral pain with right-sided sciatica. Although I was working full-time as a physical therapist, it was getting more and more difficult. This time I came down to the Institute to receive three treatments in your clinic. By the end of those sessions I was a new woman! I am pleased to report the headache, lumbosacral pain and sciatica were all gone and never returned. On top of that I could feel the uterus being derotated and it felt as if it was returned to its proper position. The pubic synthesis was opened to allow an easy delivery, which also worked. At 42-weeks gestation, I was able to deliver a 9-pound, 5-ounce baby vaginally without the use of suction, forceps, etc. I am absolutely convinced, without the cranial therapy that could not have happened.

This past year I was blessed with my second pregnancy, this one occurring the first time we tried to conceive. I was able to carry twins to 40-weeks' gestation and both were born good sizes and healthy. I did notice my son's one eye did not track and follow his other eye as he began to grow and develop. When he was one month of age, I did a cranial evaluation on him and discovered a large right temporal lesion affecting several surrounding structures, including his eye and cranial nerves. With a bit of treatment the area released and, within a short period of time, I watched the eye correct. Both eyes are now working in perfect unison. I suspect, had this problem not been corrected in the early stages of life, it would have lead to a much larger problem down the road that may have required surgery.

These are just a few of the benefits my family and I have derived from CranioSacral Therapy. The list would go on and on if I were to list them all. With healthcare reform being such a paramount issue, I truly feel CranioSacral Therapy can aid in the revolutionizing of our healthcare system.

I hope, as insurance companies work to cut costs and curtail excessive spending, that CranioSacral Therapy is seriously considered as a low-cost treatment for women during obstetrics. It certainly allowed this time in my life to be far more comfortable and enjoyable, and reduced the amount of traditional medical intervention, thus reducing suffering and cutting costs. My sincere thanks,
Pamela D. Markert, P.T.

The second letter describes a much different type of problem which was resolved as described. This writer also practices CranioSacral Therapy. I have taken editorial license with this letter in order to protect her privacy.

Dear Dr. John:

It was in the Advanced CranioSacral Therapy class that I had a wonderful experience. During the last discussion of the one week course, I remember being very restless even though I was quite sleep deprived. I remember feeling an achiness and cramps in my abdomen while trying to sit and listen attentively to everyone else's experiences.

I was waiting to tell about my SER that revisited a pregnancy I had in college which was terminated by an abortion. After all our SER discussions were completed, I went back to my room to go to the bathroom. I had had my menstrual cycle for five days and was just about finished with it. When I went to the bathroom, I passed a very large blood clot, but it did not look like a normal blood clot. At the time, the thought went through my mind that it was "the fetus" that should have been aborted 22 years ago. Of course, I have also had three live births, and a miscarriage followed by a D & C in those 22 years. This feeling of having finally aborted that fetus stayed with me. I now find that I do not have as much pain in my back and legs during my menstrual cycle, which I attribute to my SER experience. The rest of my pain during menstruation is probably left over from having had an 11-pound baby with a vaginal delivery. Maybe I'll take care of that pain next time. I find it amazing that I could experience my "reality" of having finally completed that abortion in such a very real and physical way. Thank you.

Before I close this subject, I would like to insert a description of some of the experiences that a newborn might have during a delivery process. As you read this piece, try to put yourself in the newborn's place. Now consider that most, if not all, of the residual effects of any birth experience which have registered as traumatic can be neutralized early on by appropriately applied CranioSacral Therapy and SomatoEmotional Release. It really is time to give our children the benefit of these therapeutic modalities as early in life as is possible.

Working with the newborn infant requires more from the therapist than does working with the adult. It requires more decision-making by the therapist, as well as a greater degree of self-trust. The messages from the newborn to the therapist are usually more subtle until true blending has occurred. Therefore, the therapist must sharpen his or her sensitivities, perceptual skills and, above all, he or she must blend and trust.

Think about the traumatic events that the newborn may endure during labor, delivery and post-delivery. The uterus squeezes during labor. The fetal head may be used as a "battering ram" to dilate the birth canal. This battering-ram experience may be softened by the membranes and the fluid within them. This fluid/membrane design, when it precedes the fetal head through the birth canal, serves to cushion to some extent the forces that are imposed upon the fetal head during the dilating process. But what happens when the "water" breaks spontaneously, or the membranes are ruptured deliberately by the delivery person? Woosh—there goes the "cushion," and the fetal head takes more of the brunt of the forces.

Now think about the shock it must be, not only to the physical body but also to the fetal consciousness, when hard, unbendable forceps are applied to the head, usually within the birth canal but occasionally up into the uterus when a high forceps delivery is carried out. Once applied, are the forceps placed symmetrically upon the child's head, or are they placed diagonally? If the latter is true, these forceps could most certainly induce a severe lateral strain of the cranium (sphenobasilar synchondrosis). Once in place, either correctly or incorrectly, there is always a pulling of the head, urging the rest of the body to exit the uterus. More often than not, there is also some twisting going on. The neck is most often the focus of the forces of the pull and/or twist against the resistance of the body that is being induced into the "too small" birth canal. The magnitude of the forces upon the neck and head is determined by the applied strength of the forceps operator as opposed to the size of the fetal body in relationship to the size of the birth canal. Put yourself in the place of the fetus. How does it feel? Does it feel like someone or something is wringing or even breaking your neck? Is it scary? Do you develop a few Energy Cysts, etc.?

It gets better. Consider how it feels to you, as the uninformed fetus, when someone places a "skull cap" over the crown of your presenting head. Then they turn on the vacuum/suction and start pulling you out of your mother's womb. Does it feel like someone is sucking your brains out through the soft spots in your head? Do you feel the blood, lymph, cerebrospinal fluid, neurons, soft connective tissues and even flexible bones being drawn up into the very top of your skull? What a sensation. Does it feel like you are going to die? Is the energy body being sucked up and perhaps going into the vacuum extractor? What somatoemotional, physiological, structural and energetic effects does this have on a "trusting" fetus that is already going through the somewhat scary transition from the warm, wet, rather safe womb where almost everything was furnished, to the cold, dry, harsh, bright outside world?

How about the Caesarean section (C-section)? The fetal head could be jammed into the pelvis for a long time trying unsuccessfully to dilate a birth canal which, for one reason or another, is not responding. Or a fetal butt could be stuck at the inside opening of the birth canal. How to get out? Sometimes a breech delivery is done. In the process legs are often fractured, hips dislocated, etc. More often, the C-section is done.

In the case of the jammed-in head, it often has to be pulled out of the pelvis with a "pop" very much like a cork coming out of a bottle. Imagine the sudden decompressive forces that occur when the stuck head is "popped" out of the mother's pelvis. For that matter, imagine the rapid decompressive forces to which the fetal head and body are subjected when an incision is made quickly into a uterus that is full of amniotic fluid under pressure. Sometimes this fluid squirts out of the incision a couple of inches into the air. The squirt just lasts a second or so. It's a very quick reduction of pressure upon the fetus. Would that damage your membranes? Would that cause a few capillaries to break and dump some red blood cells into the surrounding tissues? We all know that decomposing red blood cells produce bile salts. Bile salts are irritating to most tissues and will cause fibrosis to occur. When the membranes fibrose they get stiffer, and perhaps cannot accommodate the growth of the brain as readily. Brains don't do as well when they are trying to grow and develop their very complicated circuitry against restrictive pressures. How would you feel if you just went through a sudden decompression? Divers get the bends when they decompress too quickly. Sometimes they have to go into decompression chambers in order to treat the problem. Newborns have to "tough it out."

Then you are out, it is cold, the lights glare, someone is spanking you, telling you to cry and breathe. Then someone is pushing something into your mouth and perhaps down your throat a bit. That hurts some and is rather threatening. Does one of these creatures want you dead?

Those of us who have used CST-SER in obstetrical situations know that most of these traumatic situations can be corrected, neutralized, or at least the effects can be minimized when the infant is treated during the first few days after delivery. Hence, we are now offering training to CST-SER practitioners who are interested in working with pregnant women and fetuses, obstetrical deliveries and newborn infants.

The Brain Speaks

"The Brain Speaks" is the title of a new workshop that we have developed. It will continue to develop further for as long as it is presented. The seeds for "The Brain Speaks" were planted in the late 1970s and early 1980s while our clinic for brain-dysfunctioning children was in operation. It was during that time when we first became aware of the tremendous guilt that many of the parents (especially the mothers) of the afflicted children were carrying. So many of these parents felt responsible for their child's cerebral palsy, autism, seizures, dyslexia and so on. As part of our attempt to ease and/or resolve their guilt-related suffering, we developed an information booklet for parents that dealt with the intricacies of the nervous system and its development. We placed special focus upon the brain and spinal cord, and the events that were beyond the control of either parent and which might be causally related to the child's problem.

In 1993, I was prevailed upon to produce a two-part video called "A Brain Is Born," which was to be instructional for parents, caretakers and therapists who were involved with almost any type of brain-dysfunctioning child. In this video I described the development of the brain and spinal cord from conception through early childhood. I discussed several of the things that could go wrong during these times of development and functional maturation. The videos are chock-full of information. As I reviewed these videos subsequent to their final production, it became very clear to me that a written manual, which would accompany and further clarify the videos, would be helpful. I began to write this manual. One thing led to another and the "little manual" turned into a 380-page book. The publishers used large pages (8 by 11 inches) in order to keep the book from being too cumbersome in terms of its thickness. This "little manual" took me about three years to research, write and rewrite. The book is titled *A Brain Is Born*. It is a labor of love. I wrote it as simply as I could, and it crosses several interdisciplinary boundaries as it covers the formation of the sperm and the egg, the fertilization process, the development of brain and spinal cord in the uterus, and the final product. It focuses on what can go wrong, when it can go wrong, what you might see as a result of a mishap, and what can be done about it. There is also a lot of attention paid to the miracle that, considering the complexities of the developmental processes, as many things work right as they do.

As I was researching and writing this book, it became very apparent to me that there is a lot of disagreement between authorities in terms of the assigned functions of many of the brain structures and regions. There is also a vast number of unknowns which relate to brain functions, dysfunctions and the like. As I was deciphering conflicting concepts as put forth by the wide array of authorities in their various fields of expertise, I had a "eureka." Why not go to the source? In our work we "dialogue" with many internal organs, like hearts, livers, kidneys, lungs and the like. We also dialogue with the residual effects of traumatic events, whether those events are physical, as in bones, joints, muscles, etc., or emotional events, such as the loss of loved ones, physical abuse, drug abuse, etc., and/or spiritual problems. Of course, you can't prove that you have actually had a conversation with a patient's liver. But if during the conversation the cause of a liver dysfunction is elucidated and a resolution is achieved, and if after the treatment session the liver works better, whether or not you have actually spoken to the liver and its consciousness doesn't matter much (from a practical point of view). It struck me that, if we can establish a virtual rapport with a liver, why can't we do the same with the various parts of the brain?

My first real clinical experience came soon after this "eureka" had occurred. I had already had a few experiences that indicated that patients'/clients' brains could "talk" to therapists, and had begun to explore with colleagues the possibilities of dialoguing with specific brain parts. Then came a patient who had received a blow to the head with subsequent severe loss of short-term memory. She could be walking across a 20-foot room to get a book from a shelf on the other side, and en route forget which book she wanted and why. She could forget that she just ate lunch and have another lunch within an hour. We have all had episodes or experiences which we might call absent-mindedness or forgetfulness, but this woman, in her mid-40s, could not remember anything recent.

I used the CranioSacral Therapy approach to move her into a state of relaxation and altered consciousness. Had we been monitoring, I'm sure that her brain waves would have been predominantly alpha and theta. I then opened the dialogue in a friendly way and soon asked whether her brain would be willing to speak with me. A voice from within her said "yes." After a "get acquainted" conversation, I asked her brain whether there was a specific part of it that was having trouble, and whether that was the reason for the short-term memory loss. The brain's reply was that I should talk to the hippocampus (a brain structure that is understood to have a significant role in the triage of facts and/or events to be remembered). I asked if "hippocampus" would speak with me. A different-sounding inner voice answered that it would be most happy to talk to me. After some dialogue, I understood from hippocampus that it had been put into a state of "shock" during the accident because of the sudden forces that it had absorbed. In response to my further inquiries, I was led to understand that there was residual disorganized energy/force still present in hippocampus, which interfered with its ability to assign to, and retrieve from, specific brain areas the information that the patient wanted to recall. Hippocampus itself did not retain this data. Even very short-term memories were filed and retrieved from specific brain areas. It was then explained to me that I could help reorganize the energies within the hippocampus by passing my own "entraining" energies through it. If our effort at reorganization was successful, we could expect immediate restoration of short-term memory abilities. We did it with hippocampus giving feedback and guidance as we worked. At the end of the session, the patient could repeat back to me series of numbers which I gave to her verbally. She repeated back eight number series after a one-minute wait on 10 occasions with only four errors. This was quite an improvement for less than an hour's work.

The Brain Speaks workshop is aimed at helping the participant develop and use the skills necessary to carry out similar works with patients and clients. In *A Brain Is Born*, I have described over 30 different brain structures/areas. In the workshop, the participants use some of these as the focuses for beginning to learn the work. The dialogues that result seem to reveal much about these structures/areas that are either poorly understood, or about which there is little information or much disagreement. As we collect data from the workshop experiences we will begin to see experiences coming from independent sources. When similarities in function accumulate from independent dialogue experiences, we will consider these as validation and we will better understand the various functions and adaptabilities of the brain and spinal cords, as well as their many components. It is really exciting to gain this information from the source.

SomatoEmotional Release and the Psyche

I have asked a doctor of clinical psychology with more than 20 years of experience in both psychotherapy and hypnotherapy to comment upon the efficacy of SomatoEmotional Release (SER) by therapists who are not necessarily trained as psychotherapists or counselors. Russell A. Bourne, Jr., Ph.D., is that psychologist. He is familiar with the SER process and has seen it used by many therapists who are trained in CST, SER and bodywork, yet who have little or no formal training in any of the psychology-related subjects. He has seen the bodily and energetic release of emotions with only hands-on work, accompanied by some commonsense verbal support. His comments follow. We are also fortunate to have permission to reprint a short explanation of how SER is not psychotherapy, written by British osteopath John Page. His essay follows that of Dr. Bourne.

Psychology and SomatoEmotional Release by Russell A. Bourne, Jr., Ph.D.

It is with both pleasure and a bit of trepidation that I respond to John's request for a few words regarding the relationship between psychotherapy and SomatoEmotional Release. As a clinical psychologist, I am well aware of the debate concerning which professionals should provide what services in the realm of counseling and psychotherapy. Indeed, many in the varied mental health professions, i.e., psychology, psychiatry, social work and counseling, have spent hundreds of hours and thousands of pages arguing among themselves about the issue of professional competence and the appropriate limits or scope of one's practice. It seems as if many of these folks wish to equate specific academic degrees or titles with presumed competence.

I would like to explore a different set of questions in the next few pages; questions that I believe are much less controversial and fairly easily answered by professionals and laypeople alike. The first question I'd like you to consider is whether or not you believe that, in many cases, there is an emotional component to significant physical injury or disease. Most people will respond in the affirmative to this question and that, in turn, leads to a second question: Is the acknowledgment and expression of this emotional component important for healing and recovery? Nearly everyone I ask also responds with a resounding "yes." It seems quite natural to people that emotions play a major role in our health and well-being.

Now, at the risk of being pedantic, I'd like to pose two additional questions. These questions, which are also simple and straightforward, influence the nature of one's approach to healthcare. First, is it possible for a person to experience physical distress as a result of emotional or psychological causes? And second, can emotions be released through the body? Again, when I pose these questions to laypeople and professionals, the overwhelming response is something like, "Why yes, of course. Who would think otherwise?"

The idea that thoughts and emotions influence our bodies has been part of our culture and that of our ancestors for hundreds, if not thousands of years. In today's media, one can find countless references to mind/body communication and the importance of responding to the whole person when addressing matters of injury, illness or disease.

The influence of our thoughts and emotions on our bodies is quite easily demonstrated by two simple examples of ordinary human responsiveness: the act of blushing in an embarrassing situation, and the act of crying when viewing an emotional scene at the movies. In each case, an idea or thought crosses one's mind and, in a matter of seconds, the body responds. In the first case, the response is a temporary condition of localized high blood pressure in the cheeks and/or throat. In the second case, the response is the production of tears and/or the characteristic "lump" in the throat. Each of these reactions is a response to a thought—an internal process of the mind that then results directly in a physiological alteration in the body.

Now, let's return to the discussion of SomatoEmotional Release and psychotherapy. Mental health counseling and psychotherapy are respected modalities for assisting those whose lives have been affected by physical or emotional trauma, or whose progress in life has been impeded by emotional or relational conflict. There are, of course, a variety of approaches and "schools" of psychotherapy. Yet as most of you know, irrespective of theoretical orientation, counselors and psychotherapists primarily offer support, insight and understanding to those with problems. This assistance is accomplished essentially through the use of words—specific conversations and dialogue to address particular purposes or goals.

I believe strongly in the power of language, in our ability to use words and images to facilitate an alteration in perspective as well as in consciousness. Indeed, I believe language is a wonderfully effective therapeutic agent. Thus, as a psychologist who is intimately familiar with psychotherapy and SomatoEmotional Release, I wholly support the use of imagery and dialogue in the therapeutic practice of those who do CranioSacral Therapy. Since, as we've noted, language and thought influence emotions, and since emotions influence the body, it makes perfect sense to facilitate a respectful and permissive expression of that emotion, especially as it relates to the maintenance or continuation of physical distress or illness. And that, my friends, is what SomatoEmotional Release and Therapeutic Imagery and Dialogue do so well within the CranioSacral Therapy process.

Perhaps an example or two will help demonstrate the utility and individualistic quality of the SER process as practiced by Upledger-trained CranioSacral Therapists. The first case involves a woman in her late 40s who learned of The Upledger Institute, Inc., HealthPlex Clinical Services and CranioSacral Therapy while attending a support-group meeting for those with Multiple Chemical Sensitivities (MCS).

This particular patient's symptoms were diffuse and irregular. Unlike the allergy patients for whom there frequently are identifiable antagonists, either in the environment such as with mold or ragweed, or within particular food groups such as dairy or wheat products, many MCS patients are so highly reactive to their environments that it is quite difficult to identify, let alone isolate, the offending substances.

Such was the case with this patient, whose symptoms had gotten progressively worse over the prior three years. In fact, she had gotten to the point where it was necessary for her to greatly limit her daily activity, rarely leaving home, changing her clothes three or four times daily to reduce exposure and, in general, living a very narrow, isolated life. Her health was becoming increasingly compromised due to her highly restrictive diet, and the level of depression and frustration she experienced made her miserable.

After six CranioSacral Therapy treatments, she began to

venture out from the house more often and found that her energy level had improved. Yet she continued to experience feelings of depression and was very anxious about engaging in any new behavior that might cause her to have a "reaction," which was her term for the physical and emotional distress and cognitive disorientation that she experienced as a result of her MCS. Never able to predict these reactions, she became vigilant in her alertness to her environment and the potential threat that it held for her. This was contributing to a near-constant state of arousal, which was counterproductive to the goal of reducing her sensitivity.

It was during her 10th treatment session that an SER regarding this chronic state of physiological arousal and psychological tension occurred. It seemed to her that the maintenance of this hypervigilant state was necessary for her health, to keep her ever ready to protect herself from potential harm. But during the session she stated that she both needed and resented the presence of this chronic arousal. When asked to consider how she might enhance the healthfulness of this hyperaroused state while minimizing its negative influence, she was able to imagine her apprehension and tension changing to a healing energy that she could then move from her chest, face and throat areas (where she typically felt the tension) to those areas of her body that could benefit from the presence of extra support and healing. She was able to direct this healing energy to her lungs, eyes, hands and stomach over the next several weeks.

By directing the healing energy to those areas in her body that typically responded during one of her reactions, she was able to significantly reduce the frequency of reactions as well as their intensity. While she continues to be watchful of her surroundings and has yet to eliminate all chemical sensitivities, the acknowledgment of the emotional conflict she felt over her state of arousal, and the increased sense of control and interpersonal power she experienced by involving her physiology in new ways to contribute to her overall health, have contributed significantly to improving her physical well-being and quality of life.

The second case involves a woman in her late 20s who was employed as a registered nurse and had been accepted to medical school when she suffered a closed-head traumatic brain injury as a result of being hit by an automobile while riding her bike. She had completed the usual in-patient rehabilitation program at her hometown hospital before coming to the UI HealthPlex nine months after her accident.

When first seen, she was experiencing fatigue, memory loss, speech stammering, and feelings of depression and apathy—all rather typical of the myriad of post-trauma symptoms that can be experienced by patients with closed-head injuries. She had received counseling to assist her in adjusting to the reduction in her daily activity, and with the continued speech problems. By all indications, she had been a motivated and conscientious rehab patient who was working hard to regain her past abilities.

It was during her fourth CranioSacral Therapy session that a gentle inquiry was made regarding the process of her adjustment and her hopes and expectations for the future. She began to sob and expressed anger and sadness that she was not her old self, her real self. She felt betrayed by her body and did not feel that she was ever going to be the person she once was.

Of course, these feelings are quite natural for those who have experienced this level of physical trauma and loss of abilities. Yet before this session, she had not been able to actively state her feelings of loss, disappointment and frustration.

Indeed, she had not permitted herself to grieve for the loss of her "whole self," and the emotional energy spent containing these feelings of grief and sadness had been significant. It seemed that she had maintained an extreme state of physical tension in her effort to control the expression of these emotions. Consequently, this physical tension had interrupted her normal speech pattern. Additionally, her preoccupation with her "old self" and the near obsessive orientation to the past had served to fuel her depression and interrupt her movement toward recovery.

As she was allowed to release the grief of her lost self, she released the physical tension throughout her mouth, jaw, throat and thoracic inlet. At the end of the session, she and her companion were equally surprised by the degree of immediate improvement in her speech. She stammered less frequently and her thoughts flowed more freely. Throughout the next several sessions she continued to improve in both speech, cognition and mood.

At the conclusion of her visit, she stated that she had found a way to say good-bye to her old self and was encouraged by the process of beginning to get to know her new self. Her gains from CranioSacral Therapy and SomatoEmotional Release were clearly physical and psychological. With the absence of the barriers that were inherent in her earlier state of repressed grief and sadness, she had progressed to a place of greater physical well-being and renewed optimism.

In both of these cases, there were physical and emotional restrictions. When released, these interferences manifested as detectable physical energy. The rationale of a physical energetic presence before and after physical trauma follows a commonsense logic. A bit more surprising was the realization of a physical energy response to the emotional aspects of illness and injury. Yet, as I mentioned at the beginning of these remarks, the manner in which emotions may influence our bodies is profound. Since the body's response system is essentially energetic (i.e., biochemical, electromagnetic and vibrational), it makes perfect sense that an emotional release may be accompanied by a significant release of felt energy.

In the first case, the perception of this energy was combined with a perceptible rise in body temperature over a localized area in the patient's chest. Heat seemed to emanate from just above her sternum for approximately 60 seconds, and was followed by a very deep and prolonged vocal sigh. It was as if she had released a tremendous burdensome energy held tightly within her upper body.

In the second case, a spasm-like vibration within the patient's neck and shoulders occurred simultaneously with the felt sense of a magnetic force pushing the therapist's hands off the patient's body. This palpable energy phenomenon lasted for 20 to 30 seconds and, as in the case of the first patient, also resulted in an audible and deeply resonant sigh of release.

As John has written elsewhere, the release of these Energy Cysts seems to permit a reorganization within the body/mind/spirit complex of each patient. The personal resources once needed to contain these respective cysts of energy are no longer needed to preserve a dysfunctional status quo. Thus, the patient's healing can now move forward in more appropriate ways.

The benefits of combining SomatoEmotional Release and Therapeutic Imagery and Dialogue with the therapeutic techniques of CranioSacral Therapy are without question. The body, mind and spirit are one when it comes to promoting the realization of the full potential of each of us and, quite obviously, the health of any one of these dimensions influences the health of the others.

As my doctoral chairman at the University of Virginia, Dr.

Paul Walter, taught me years ago, "What we are to be, we are always becoming." This respect for our individual developmental process is characteristic of the principles of CranioSacral Therapy and SomatoEmotional Release. Furthermore, John Upledger's recognition of the developmental process of ideas and shifting paradigms, as well as the innovations they suggest, sets him apart from most in our professions. Indeed, it benefits all of us when individuals such as Dr. Upledger continue to investigate approaches to healthcare designed to assist each of us in our personal journey toward health and well-being, toward realizing our full potential and becoming all that we can be in this lifetime.

How is SER Not Psychotherapy? by John Page, D.O.
SER involves physical contact, physical process. It is essentially a physical therapy involving the thought processes, the awareness. Psychology requires no physical contact or process. Psychotherapy applies itself to a previously identified task using pre-ordained tools. SER is a shared adventure, ideally not pre-arranged, that thrives on the unexpected. SER requires the flexible use of many tools, and continues to invent new ones, presenting them as gifts to the aware and flexible facilitator. Psychotherapy is directed by a knowledgeable expert. SER is helped by a facilitator, part of whose skill is not to need to know what's there.

Psychotherapy has systems, traditions, approaches and specialties. Thus we have Rebirthers, Past Life therapists, etc. The patient is a person-in-need, disempowered, who is seeking help from an outside expert. There can be temptation for the patient to perform, to fit in with the psychotherapist by supporting his or her belief system. SER has no system as such. Psychotherapy can be used symptomatically, like a Band-Aid®. SER aims at releasing causes.

Psychotherapy is done by one person to another, in much the same way that physiotherapy is applied. SER is done by the person, for themselves with the help of others.

SER can happen spontaneously.

26

Questions & Answers

Pregnancy & Obstetrics

Q Is it safe for me to have CranioSacral Therapy now that I'm pregnant?

A: Yes, it is safe, and even desirable, because CranioSacral Therapy mobilizes and enhances many of the normal adaptational processes of your body. It is necessary for these processes to be highly operative during pregnancy. CranioSacral Therapy can very definitely assist them.

Q: I heard that CranioSacral Therapy can induce labor. Will it induce labor prematurely?

A: CranioSacral Therapy assists normal physiological processes. When properly applied it will never go against what your body wants to do. Therefore, it will never induce premature labor unless there is something wrong with the pregnancy and your body naturally wants to abort the fetus.

Q: If my labor seems to be going nowhere, can CranioSacral Therapy help me?

A: Yes, CranioSacral Therapy often seems to be the vehicle

that puts energy into a stalled labor. This may happen by many different mechanisms, but it doesn't really matter which is theoretically correct. CranioSacral Therapy is often followed by a quick natural delivery.

Newborns & Infants

Q: How soon can a newborn child be treated with CranioSacral Therapy?
A: Depending upon the skill of the CranioSacral Therapist, the first treatment could be done within minutes of the obstetrical delivery. The younger the newborn, the more skilled the therapist must be. The craniosacral system's activity is extremely subtle at the time of delivery, but becomes more apparent as the hours of life outside the womb go by. In order to be sure of what he/she is doing, the CranioSacral Therapist should be able to perceive the craniosacral rhythm of the newborn. So for one therapist, one hour after delivery may be the right time to treat the child. Another therapist with less experience and perceptual development may need to wait a day, a week, a month or a year.

Q: Why would I want my newborn child treated?
A: CranioSacral Therapy can correct problems in the craniosacral system immediately and permanently. These problems, when corrected, may avoid the development of colic, respiratory problems, hyperactivity, dyslexia, seizure disorders, floppy baby syndrome and allergies. Although not proven as yet, I believe it can also thwart many cases of cerebral palsy, scoliosis, and dental problems that require orthodontia later in life. Furthermore, it has been shown that the child's general health is improved.

Postpartum Mothers

Q: How can CranioSacral Therapy help the new mother?
A: In several ways: (1) It helps restore hormone balance; (2) It helps alleviate postpartum depression; and (3) It restores normal pelvic function, thus eliminating many post-delivery back problems and the like.

Q: I had problems with high blood pressure after my second delivery. Could CranioSacral Therapy help this?
A: Very often high blood pressure for any reason returns to normal after just a few CranioSacral Therapy sessions.

Q: How about helping me lose the weight gained during pregnancy?
A: If normalizing your endocrine system and mobilizing your bodily fluids would help you lose weight, the answer is yes.

Children

Q: What kinds of problems with children does CranioSacral Therapy help?
A: This is a tremendously broad question. I'll try to answer it based only on my own personal experience.
   1. *Allergies*
   Respiratory—CranioSacral Therapy is very definitely helpful when combined with SomatoEmotional Release.
   Food—CranioSacral Therapy is also helpful when structural problems of the skull are found and released. There are other reasons for food allergies that are not necessarily affected by CranioSacral Therapy.
   2. *Colic, digestive and elimination problems* are corrected by

CranioSacral Therapy about 75 percent of the time unless they are due to tumors or other significant pathological problems.

3. *Psychological problems*—CranioSacral Therapy helps the therapist develop trust and rapport with the child very quickly. In this way the emotional problems can be discovered. On the other hand, I have seen several "psychological" problems disappear when a craniosacral problem was corrected. These problems had no emotional basis. Although they appeared to be psychological, they were due to physiological craniosacral system dysfunction.

4. *Hyperactive children* are very effectively treated by Cranio-Sacral Therapy when the problem is not emotional in origin. In my experience, about 50 to 60 percent of hyperactive child problems have a basis in the craniosacral system.

5. *Learning disabilities and dyslexia*—As in the case of hyperactive children, when the problem originates in the craniosacral system, the treatment is very effective. This is about 50 to 60 percent of the time.

6. *Down's syndrome*—This is a very difficult question. What I can say is that Down's syndrome children who have received CranioSacral Therapy have been happy and often exceeded conventional expectations.

7. *Mental retardation*—Whether or not the "retarded" child will respond dramatically to CranioSacral Therapy depends upon the cause for the "retardation." I have had some remarkably positive results in selected cases. In others, they got healthier when treated, but didn't necessarily get smarter.

8. *Cerebral palsy*—Most of my experience has been with spastic cases. These children have all improved—some very dramatically, some just a little. Once again, it depends on

the cause of the palsy. Sometimes the spasticity is relieved but the child is left with flaccid paralysis. Flaccid is more comfortable than spastic, so this is worth something.

9. *Seizures*—The response of the seizure-disordered child is strictly dependent upon the reason for the seizures. I have seen many children completely stop having seizures with no medication as the CranioSacral Therapy was carried out. Some children whose seizures are due to deeper brain disorders do not respond at all. The majority stop having seizures and require a reduced dosage of medication.

10. *Autism*—We did three years of intensive research with autistic children in the late 1970s. We saw significant improvement in self-destructive behavior, in the display of affection, and in social interaction. These improvements usually deteriorated within three to six months after CranioSacral Therapy was discontinued. This is an ideal situation for parents to learn to treat their child, and a matter for further research.

Q: Does CranioSacral Therapy provide any benefit for the normal child?
A: I feel very strongly that CranioSacral Therapy is one of the more powerful and effective health-enhancement treatment programs available today. So in view of my bias, the answer is yes.

Q: I heard that CranioSacral Therapy can be used in childhood diseases like measles, mumps, chicken pox, etc.
A: My experience has been that CranioSacral Therapy can be used to effectively break the fever and ease the child through the crisis in most of these conditions. I think it bolsters the immune system and mobilizes the autonomic nervous system so that the body's defenses are better used.

Q: What about scoliosis?
A: In some cases of scoliosis, the cause is craniosacral. More often than not, though, the tube of dura mater membrane that goes down the spinal canal has a twist/torque in it that can be detected very early in life. The spine resists the torque as long as it can, but sometime in the prepubescent period or in early adolescence, the spine begins to twist in response to the twisted dura mater membrane. This is the beginning of a scoliosis. Sometimes, if caught early, this can be corrected using CranioSacral Therapy, and the scoliosis disappears.

Q: How does CranioSacral Therapy work with orthodontia?
A: Very well indeed. It often shortens the course of orthodontia and occasionally eliminates the need entirely. I suggest that all children have CranioSacral Therapy before embarking on a course of orthodontic correction.

Q: Can you help cross-eyed children?
A: When the problem is due to dura mater membrane tension affecting the nerves to the eyes, the results are excellent and dramatic. I have helped several children avoid eye surgery using CranioSacral Therapy techniques.

Adults

Q: I don't really have a complaint, but I am curious. Could I get CranioSacral Therapy?
A: By all means. We really believe that CranioSacral Therapy on a regular basis, no matter how good you feel, is some of the best health-enhancement activity that you can do. You

may discover that you feel even better than you thought you could. I'm sure that you will have fewer sick days.

Q: What does CranioSacral Therapy do for headaches?
A: Headaches are one of the most common complaints that we treat with CranioSacral Therapy and its offshoots. I would say that we are 80 to 90 percent successful no matter what type of headache is presented to us.

Q: How about chronic back pain?
A: Once again, the success is outstanding when CranioSacral Therapy is used for back pain, including ruptured discs. We work from the inside ("core") out. When the "core" is corrected, the outside (peripheral problem) either corrects itself or becomes amenable to conventional treatment.

Q: I heard that you offer special intensive programs through your clinic in Florida. What are they and how do they work?
A: A number of one- and two-week intensive programs are offered through our UI HealthPlex clinic in Palm Beach Gardens, Florida. Among the conditions addressed are: brain and spinal cord dysfunction, learning disabilities, post-traumatic stress, autism, pain, cancer recovery and therapist rejuvenation. Each program features a specially selected team of clinicians comprised of UI HealthPlex staff and skilled visiting therapists. Drawing on a variety of complementary approaches, including CranioSacral Therapy and Somato-Emotional Release, the clinicians work together in multiple-hands sessions as needed to address the specific health concerns of each individual. These programs offer an

exceptional opportunity to receive some of the most innovative healthcare currently available anywhere. For information, you can call the clinic at 561-622-4706.

Q: If this treatment method is so good, why isn't it incorporated into the conventional healthcare system?
A: Change takes time. More and more recognition is coming our way, but we are flying in the face of many dogmas, not the least of which are:
1. Skull bones don't move.
2. Minds can't control bodies.
3. All memory is in the brain.
4. Transference of energy between patient and therapist is ridiculous.
5. Nervous-tissue injury is permanent.
And so on...
In view of these antiquated but firmly held beliefs, I think our level of acceptance is remarkably good.

Q: What can you do for depression?
A: In specific types of depression, CranioSacral Therapy is probably the most effective treatment available. In others, when combined with SomatoEmotional Release and Therapeutic Imagery and Dialogue, the results are good.

Q: What can you do for PMS?
A: In most cases we can move the patient toward total eradication of this problem. CranioSacral Therapy can and does help the pelvic organs to function more efficiently. We also improve the function of the endocrine system—in this case the pituitary, adrenal and ovarian glands.

Q: What about chronic fluid retention? Can you help that?
A: CranioSacral Therapy enhances fluid mobility throughout the body; therefore it helps fluid retention, whether due to heart problems, kidney problems, mineral imbalance, or any other cause. It must be done regularly if the cause is ongoing. Here we like to teach a family member or loved one to treat the patient on a daily basis.

Q: What is your track record with arthritis?
A: There are several kinds of arthritis. The most common is osteoarthritis. Probably the most notorious is rheumatoid, which is inflammatory in nature. Both types of arthritis are amenable and responsive to CranioSacral Therapy. In these cases we also like to teach family members to treat the patient daily. This approach gives the best response.

Q: I hear you have had some interesting results with coma patients.
A: Yes, the number of patients is not high, but of the few I've treated the results have ranged from good to spectacular. Some of our more advanced students report similar results. We would welcome the opportunity to do more work in this field.

Q: What's the difference between CranioSacral Therapy, Cranial Osteopathy, Chiropractic Craniopathy and Sacro-Occipital Technique?
A: In the other approaches mentioned above, the movement of the bones is the major objective. In CranioSacral Therapy, bones are used to manipulate much more deeply into the system of membranes and fluids. Therefore the bone movement is an enabling objective in CranioSacral Therapy. In all fair-

ness, the other forms of cranial work are beginning to use the concepts of CranioSacral Therapy and are starting to look and work more deeply now.

Another major difference is that CranioSacral Therapy uses a much lighter touch. Most often, the patient's internal forces and energies provide what is required for therapeutic corrections of the craniosacral system.

In cranial work, as practiced in both the traditional osteopathic and chiropractic modes, the therapist more often than not forces the "correction" upon the patient. This approach allows for more mistakes by the therapist and for more trauma to result from the treatment sessions.

Q: Why do some people feel worse after a treatment?
A: There are several reasons for this post-treatment discomfort. One is that their body is re-experiencing a previous trauma or injury as it is releasing from the tissues. This can take a few days. Another is that areas of "numbness" have come back to "life" and are more sensitive. Also, it often happens that the body has adapted to a malfunction. When we remove the adaptation as we get closer to the nucleus of the problem, the suppressed pain comes back to the surface.

We must also consider that pain is a perception. When hope of correction of a problem is held out before the patient, the nonconscious makes the pain worse so that we won't stop before the whole problem is solved. There are many more individual reasons for a worsening of symptoms after a good treatment.

We cannot neglect the possibility that the therapist screwed up. This can cause a painful reaction. This screw-up is usually by the application of excessive force and/or trying to make the patient's body do what the therapist decides is right. We preach the sermon of "follow the body, don't lead it."

Q: What is tissue or cell memory?
A: I don't know exactly, but if you watch what happens during treatment and healing processes, it looks like individual tissues and probably cells have recall of experiences they have gone through.

Q: How can you tell what is wrong with me by picking up my legs?
A: We use the perception of very subtle energy activities in the body to focus on the source of abnormal energy patterns. We also very gently traction the legs to see if resistance of tissues is equal or lacks symmetry. We do these kinds of evaluations all over your body; you just notice it more in your legs because picking up the legs is more apparent to you than when we touch your ribs, your shoulders or your head. But we are doing essentially the same kind of evaluation on many body regions.

Q: Why does it look like the therapist isn't moving?
A: Because we are just barely moving. What we look for in CranioSacral Therapy is extremely subtle. It takes practice, but once learned you have it forever.

Q: How can you get any treatment done using such a light touch?
A: As I said earlier, in CranioSacral Therapy we try very hard to get the patient's body to make the correction. We, the therapists, assist the natural corrective tendency of the patient's body. When you use more than a little force, you may recruit the patient's bodily defense against your intrusion. When the patient's body begins to defend itself against the therapist, the tissues of the patient's body tighten in an attempt to preserve the status quo. When confronted with this situation, the therapist can: (1) apply more force to overcome patient resis-

tance; or (2) lighten up the touch, as we do in CranioSacral Therapy, thus allowing the patient's tissues to relax and obtaining a therapeutic release by adding just enough to the patient's own self-corrective mechanism to be effective.

Once again we are confronted with that difference in approach which separates CranioSacral Therapy from other cranial techniques. This difference is what makes Cranio-Sacral Therapy so safe and so useable by non-physicians. It can be applied cookbook style and still obtain an excellent therapeutic result.

Q: I've had CranioSacral Therapy, and I was astonished by the approach. My pain was in my shoulder, and it was cured by the therapist working with my sacrum and pelvis. How can this happen?

A: There are several possible ways this could happen. First, the craniosacral system connects the sacrum and pelvis to the neck and head via the tube of dura mater membrane that runs through the spinal canal. An abnormal tension on this membrane at the tail end can easily show up at the head end. In this case the abnormal membrane tension probably was just right to pull on the membrane sleeves that cover the nerve roots as they go out to the shoulder. This pull would make a perception of pain where the nerve root goes, in this case to your shoulder.

Another possibility depends upon the head-to-tail continuity of the connective tissue (fascia) that ensheathes all muscles, bones, organs, etc. A twist in the pelvis could easily ascend your body outside of the craniosacral system through this fascia to the fascia and/or the nerves to your shoulder.

Yet another possibility is that the sacrum was twisted and causing a twist to go up the total spine in a compensatory way. If there is a little less tolerance in the openings where nerve roots pass out of the spinal canal between the vertebrae in your lower neck, the nerve to your shoulder could get pinched. In any of these cases, when the abnormal situation in the sacrum and pelvis is corrected, the effect up high in the neck is removed and the pain goes away.

It takes a good therapist to find the cause at such distances. In teaching CranioSacral Therapy we put a lot of time and effort into teaching whole-body diagnosis. This approach uncovers the underlying cause, even at such distances from the pain.

Q: Why do I have a TMJ problem when there is nothing wrong with my teeth?

A: The TMJ problem, in my experience, is more often an effect or result of craniosacral system or muscle-bone-joint system dysfunction. I described one case for you where the TMJ problem came from the muscles of the buttocks. You are a whole person, and every part of you is connected to every other part. We can't let pain and symptom location mislead us. Find the cause. It may be well camouflaged. It may be located almost anywhere, but its discovery is part of the joy of doing this work.

Q: Does CranioSacral Therapy help those of us who are getting older, stiffer, more fragile and losing our memories?

A: The answer is a resounding "Yes." I have treated people regularly who are well into their 80s. These people get more agile and mobile. They get more energy and show improved intellect and memory. It also helps fight fluid retention and improves resistance to colds, flu, etc.

Q: How can older folks best use CranioSacral Therapy?

A: Ideally I would like to see the elderly patient treated once a month by a competent CranioSacral Therapist. In addition, I would like to see family members trained in some very simple techniques so that they can apply limited CranioSacral Therapy to those elderly folks at least three times per week. I have successfully taught elderly people to treat each other on occasion. This imparts a wonderful boost to the treater's sense of self-worth.

Incidentally, our success using specific and very easy-to-learn CranioSacral Therapy techniques for small-stroke patients has been excellent.

Q: How can I get treated by a CranioSacral Therapist?
A: We have several highly qualified people at our Upledger Institute, Inc., HealthPlex Clinical Services in Palm Beach Gardens, Florida, who would be happy to see you and introduce you to our approach. You can reach them at 561-622-4706. We also offer an alumni directory composed of licensed healthcare practitioners who have taken the postgraduate courses in CranioSacral Therapy. You can purchase this directory through The Upledger Institute at 1-800-233-5880, or locally at 561-622-4334.

Q: What are the credentials of those you refer outside the Institute?
A: While we're cautious about referrals due to legal ramifications, we'll guide you to people who have satisfactorily completed our own advanced program. Our only requirement is that they have a license to practice in a healthcare profession that legally allows them to do CranioSacral Therapy. We will guide you to someone who has demonstrated good skills in the use of CranioSacral Therapy. That person could be a medical doctor, an osteopathic physician, a dentist, a chiropractor,

a registered nurse, a physical therapist, an occupational therapist, a massage therapist, a Rolfer, a Soma practitioner, another type of bodyworker, or an acupuncturist. We even have a few psychotherapists who have taken up our work and become very proficient with their hands. The main issue is their hands-on skill. We will tell you about their other credentials, and you have to decide whether or not you find that person acceptable to see for CranioSacral Therapy.

Q: Does insurance pay for CranioSacral Therapy?
A: The best answer I can give you is that it depends on the credentials of the therapist and upon the extent and scope of your coverage. We are gaining more and more recognition for CranioSacral Therapy from insurance companies, but change does not occur overnight. This is very new stuff we're doing. The results will ultimately be the vehicle whereby recognition is obtained.

Q: How can I help support the work of The Upledger Institute?
A: The Upledger Foundation is our non-profit division responsible for the continued research and development of new techniques along with providing financial assistance to many patients who require intensive therapy. It is a charitable organization under section 501(c)(3) of the internal revenue code. Tax-deductible donations may be sent to:

The Upledger Foundation
11211 Prosperity Farms Road
Palm Beach Gardens, FL 33410-3487

Closing
I hope that this book has opened some doors for you. I also hope that you get some of your power back. After all, we were

all born with the power to help heal each other. Then we were convinced that we couldn't do it. Try it, you can do it.

Remember, CranioSacral Therapy, Tissue Memory, Energy Cyst Release, Direction of Energy, SomatoEmotional Release and Therapeutic Imagery and Dialogue are all very natural approaches to health and healing. If done with reasonable common sense, any or all of them are virtually without risk of side effect. Few therapeutic approaches can make this claim.

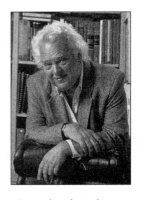

Dr. John E. Upledger (D.O., O.M.M., D.Sc.) is a Certified Fellow of the American Academy of Osteopathy, an Academic Fellow of the British Society of Osteopathy, and Doctor of Science. His specialties include Osteopathic Manipulation, CranioSacral Therapy, Somato-Emotional Release®, Acupuncture, and Preventative Medicine. Throughout Dr. Upledger's career as an osteopathic physician, he has been recognized as an innovator and leading proponent in the investigation of new therapies. His development of CranioSacral Therapy, in particular, has gained him an international reputation.

Although much of his experience was garnered through private clinical practice, Dr. Upledger served from 1975-1983 as a clinical researcher and professor of biomechanics at Michigan State University. It was during those years that he supervised a team of anatomists, physiologists, biophysicists and bioengineers in experiments testing the existence and influence of the craniosacral system. As a result of their scientific studies, the function of the craniosacral system and its use in evaluating and treating poorly understood malfunctions of the brain and spinal cord were explained. It was also during this time that Dr. Upledger developed and refined the techniques of CranioSacral Therapy which today are taught through the Upledger Institute's educational program to a diversified group of healthcare professionals, including osteopathic physicians, medical doctors, psychiatrists, dentists, nurses, chiropractors, physical therapists, occupational therapists, and massage therapists.

Dr. Upledger's books include *CranioSacral Therapy, CranioSacral Therapy II: Beyond the Dura, SomatoEmotional Release and Beyond,* and *A Brain is Born.*